Recurrent Spontaneous Miscarriages

Recurrent Spontaneous Miscarriages

Third Edition

Pankaj Desai MD FICOG FICMCH
Consultant and Specialist
Obstetrics and Gynecology
Janani Maternity Hospital
Vadodara, Gujarat, India

Formerly

Dean of Students
Medical College
Vadodara, Gujarat, India

Associate Professor and Unit Chief
Department of Obstetrics and Gynecology
Medical College and SSG Hospital
Vadodara, Gujarat, India

President
Federation of Obstetric and Gynaecological
Societies of India (FOGSI), 2007

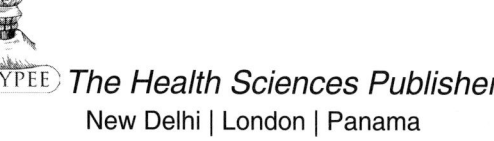

JAYPEE *The Health Sciences Publisher*
New Delhi | London | Panama

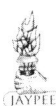 **Jaypee Brothers Medical Publishers (P) Ltd**

Headquarters
Jaypee Brothers Medical Publishers (P) Ltd.
4838/24, Ansari Road, Daryaganj
New Delhi 110 002, India
Phone: +91-11-43574357
Fax: +91-11-43574314
E-mail: jaypee@jaypeebrothers.com

Overseas Offices

JP Medical Ltd.
83, Victoria Street, London
SW1H 0HW (UK)
Phone: +44-20 3170 8910
Fax: +44(0)20 3008 6180
E-mail: info@jpmedpub.com

Jaypee-Highlights Medical Publishers Inc.
City of Knowledge, Bld. 235, 2nd Floor, Clayton
Panama City, Panama
Phone: +1 507-301-0496
Fax: +1 507-301-0499
E-mail: cservice@jphmedical.com

Jaypee Brothers Medical Publishers (P) Ltd.
17/1-B, Babar Road, Block-B, Shyamoli
Mohammadpur, Dhaka-1207
Bangladesh
Mobile: +08801912003485
E-mail: jaypeedhaka@gmail.com

Jaypee Brothers Medical Publishers (P) Ltd.
Bhotahity, Kathmandu, Nepal
Phone: +977-9741283608
E-mail: kathmandu@jaypeebrothers.com

Website: www.jaypeebrothers.com
Website: www.jaypeedigital.com

© 2018, Jaypee Brothers Medical Publishers

The views and opinions expressed in this book are solely those of the original contributor(s)/author(s) and do not necessarily represent those of editor(s) of the book.

All rights reserved. No part of this publication may be reproduced, stored or transmitted in any form or by any means, electronic, mechanical, photocopying, recording or otherwise, without the prior permission in writing of the publishers.

All brand names and product names used in this book are trade names, service marks, trademarks or registered trademarks of their respective owners. The publisher is not associated with any product or vendor mentioned in this book.

Medical knowledge and practice change constantly. This book is designed to provide accurate, authoritative information about the subject matter in question. However, readers are advised to check the most current information available on procedures included and check information from the manufacturer of each product to be administered, to verify the recommended dose, formula, method and duration of administration, adverse effects and contraindications. It is the responsibility of the practitioner to take all appropriate safety precautions. Neither the publisher nor the author(s)/editor(s) assume any liability for any injury and/or damage to persons or property arising from or related to use of material in this book.

This book is sold on the understanding that the publisher is not engaged in providing professional medical services. If such advice or services are required, the services of a competent medical professional should be sought.

Every effort has been made where necessary to contact holders of copyright to obtain permission to reproduce copyright material. If any have been inadvertently overlooked, the publisher will be pleased to make the necessary arrangements at the first opportunity. The **CD/DVD-ROM** (if any) provided in the sealed envelope with this book is complimentary and free of cost. **Not meant for sale.**

Inquiries for bulk sales may be solicited at: jaypee@jaypeebrothers.com

Recurrent Spontaneous Miscarriages

First Edition: 2009
Second Edition: 2014
Third Edition: **2018**
ISBN: 978-93-5270-276-3
Printed at: Sanat Printers

Preface to the Third Edition

I never expected that in less than 5 years, 4 to be precise, this book would warrant one more edition. It shows the popularity and usefulness this book enjoys. Before I started writing this edition, I sent nearly 25,000 emails to its potential readers all over inviting their suggestions. Many of them sent very 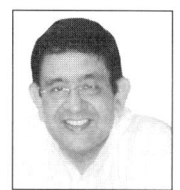 valuable inputs. I have tried to incorporate nearly all, which has fortified this edition and has made it more reader-relevant.

As I had mentioned in the previous edition, this book is a part of my study of the subject of immunology in obstetrics of last three decades. I have always felt that as a teacher and as a scientist it is the responsibility of our community to share what all we learn and gain. Writing such books is a part of that sharing process. Paulo Coelho has said "Writing means sharing. It is part of the human condition to want to share things-thoughts, ideas, and opinions". Though this is the third edition with the current publisher, I had also published a book titled "Recurrent Miscarriage more than a decade ago, as the first in this series. One can therefore, take the liberty of calling this as the fourth edition. Incessant advances in the field, necessitated a periodic overhaul and so editions after editions followed.

In the present edition, I have incorporated many nuances. The most prominent of these is the importance of color Doppler in the management of subjects with recurrent spontaneous miscarriages. One of the commonest causes of recurrent miscarriages is immunological vasculopathy. Vasculopathies have a vascular basis and so it is pertinent to view what is happening within the vessels. Color Doppler does precisely this. Once, I started going into the depth of the vascular basis of recurrent miscarriages, I found an entire new world opening up. Though it is intriguing, it also gave many solutions. It can reveal that the process of vasculopathy is active in any indexed pregnancy. At the same time, it can also predict a possible outcome. I have included this in great details in the book.

Charged with the information provided by color Doppler, we as obstetricians are able to take decisive steps of preventive measures. As one of the earliest proponent of the use of heparin in recurrent spontaneous miscarriages of immunological origin, I always wanted a tool to help me in deciding in which subjects I can discontinue using heparin, earlier. Previously, before using color Doppler so extensively, we used to continue using heparin till 36 weeks of pregnancy and after stopping for a week induce labor at 37 weeks. Thanks to this new technology I am now able to discontinue Heparin much earlier. This aspect gets a detailed discussion in the pages to follow.

All these results had to pass through a rigorous statistical scrutiny. Many of these results have been published in peer-reviewed journals. I did not confine it only to the Chi-square test but also used other statistical tests to fortify the validity of these results. Only when more than one statistical tool indicated that one particular result was scientifically valid, would then I take a stand on its efficacy. Some results were statistically untenable and therefore mercilessly rejected. It was an exercise of revelation and development.

It is with a great sense of satisfaction that I have to report to the readers that results corroborating ours, regarding the use of low-dose aspirin, have started trickling in from around the world, of late. However, Indian obstetricians (on the basis of very solid scientific results published) are using low-dose aspirin for more than two decades. The world just follows!

Ultrasound, in general, is the most important aid for an obstetrician when one has to handle subjects with recurrent spontaneous miscarriages. I have covered this aspect in details. Also, there is a continuous support taken of this technology in specific chapters like "Anatomical causes of Recurrent Spontaneous Miscarriages."

Genetics is a maze, more so when it comes to recurrent miscarriages. As in the previous edition, we have renowned geneticist Dr. Sharad Gogate to pen this chapter. He is the only contributing author in this book. He has thoroughly revised his chapter, making it updated.

Evidence-based practice is a wonderful lamp which decisively breaks down the darkness of unscientific approaches including recurrent spontaneous miscarriages. When I was updating this chapter, I was delighted as any scientist should be. There were many aspects which may have been held valid previously, now not found to be valid anymore. There were others that were reinforced and evidence for some new aspects seeped in into the scene. Updating this chapter, therefore, was a greatly illuminating exercise.

Reproduction has a strong endocrinal basis. Some of the reproductive hormones have been found to have an immunological face. While updating the chapter on the endocrinology of recurrent spontaneous miscarriages I thoroughly examined the latest evidence to take a stand. Progesterone and human chorionic gonadotropin (hCG) were always eyed with suspicion for their efficacy in preventing recurrent miscarriages. There was such a wide gap between the clinical use of these hormones as supplements and their efficacy. Thankfully some evidence has appeared showing that they may, after all, be effective. However to what extent is this efficacy valid, remains a mystery. Maybe in subsequent editions, I may get evidence to bridge the yawning chasm between evidence and the mighty use of these agents in clinical practice.

Many interesting developments are now on the horizon spelling out the importance of sonographic imaging of the cervix in pregnancy. This has made the use of cervical cerclage much more accurate and scientific. It has reduced the need for this invasive procedure remarkably in practice. This aspect also has been dealt with in detail in this new edition. Cervical cerclage versus progesterone supplementation is a new debate on the horizon. As a scientist, I have always felt that cervical cerclage may be an overused procedure. Now with progesterone walking down the hall holding the banner that it can completely replace cerclage, it became necessary for me to visit this controversy. Have I found the answer?—well not a complete one! The truth lies midway.

Why do I retain endometriosis and infections in this book, editions after editions? The answer is plain and simple—many clinicians still continue to pay obeisance to these two as important causes of recurrent spontaneous miscarriages. Ten years down the line and more, science has found no credible evidence to associate any of these with recurrent miscarriages. Until that time the requesting investigations for TORCH in particular and infections, in general, continues to be scribbled by practitioners of our subject and I will be including these in the book.

So as to make this edition free of grammatical mistakes and free of spelling errors, I have purchased the use of two softwares, besides getting the manuscript checked by a competent copy-editor. I assure you, I have done the best for this. However, if some errors may have still crept passed the scrutinizing eyes of the checking systems please ignore them.

I have tried to make this monogram as comprehensive as possible. However, I know that this is not the final word on recurrent spontaneous miscarriages as yet. New knowledge will continue to flow in, new research with continue to be game-changers and new technology will continue to change our approach to the subject. I will continue working in this field inspired by one of the greatest Indian rishis of modern times, Dr. A. P. J. Kalam who said "Never stop fighting until you arrive at your destined place - that is, the unique you. Have an aim in life, continuously acquire knowledge, work hard, and have the perseverance to realize the great life."

In all humility, I place this book in the hands of the keen students of our subject (as clinicians, postgraduate students or research scientists) hoping to get their blessings in my pursuit of academic excellence at the service of humanity and mankind.

17th January 2018

Pankaj Desai
Vadodara, India

Preface to the First Edition

Recurrent Spontaneous Miscarriages, as they are popularly called, touch a vast canvas from immunology to psychology. No wonder, it will have many facets and bearings. At the same time, with the science of obstetrics making giant strides due to influx of modern technology, the face of this entity is bound to change. My forays to understand this clinical condition is now more than two decades old. It all began with an unassuming question on this problem that I tossed to a PG student once during a teaching session and her failure to answer, made me start studying this challenge in depth. It was after assiduously following subjects of recurrent spontaneous miscarriages that I realized its links with seemingly diverse conditions like PIH, accidental hemorrhage, IUGR and recurrent stillbirths.

Once, we had the facility for testing of antiphospholipid antibodies at Vadodara during which our search for the causes and treatment became more productive and much water has flown under the bridge since then. I studied many research papers and chapters in different books later, and I am now fascinated by the advent of Color Doppler and 4-D Imaging Techniques on this subject.

In this book, I have invited two meritorious and knowledgeable authors Dr Sharad Gogate (Chapter 5) and Dr Jayakrishnan (Chapter 3) to share their expertise in the fields of chromosomal and anatomical cause of recurrent spontaneous miscarriages. Like immunological causes these need very special skills and experience to handle them. I am very thankful to them for their contributions.

I would be failing in my duty if I do not thank my wife Dr Meera Desai and my children Ushma and Shlok for their support during the completion of this book project.

My typist and loyalist for nearly 20 years, Mr Ramesh Kadam needs a special pat on his back. Though a graduate in arts for whom medical jargon could be perplexing, he deftly typed the manuscript reasonably flawlessly and shared this load mightily with me.

Before I place this book in the hands of the readers, I would like to pray to Goddess Aetheus (Maa Saraswati) of knowledge to make this book valid so that the knowledge that flows here may help the reader handle patients of recurrent spontaneous miscarriages scientifically. This will ultimately help us serve humanity and mankind better.

Pankaj Desai

Acknowledgments

Brené Brown, a renowned research professor at the University of Houston, has beautifully said, "I don't have to chase extraordinary moments to find happiness—it is right in front of me, if I am paying attention and practicing gratitude." As I place third edition of this book in your hands, I would like to express my heartfelt gratitude to all those who have directly or indirectly helped me.

First of all, I express my gratitude to all my readers who have given me so many blessings, support, and encouragement that this book has gone into its new edition in a short span of time. I feel overwhelmed by their kindness.

I would also like to offer my thanks to Dr Sharad Gogate. He has kindly authored chapter *Genetics of Recurrent Miscarriages and Other Pregnancy Losses*, in this edition as well. He is the Director, Surlata Hospital and Fetal Medicine Consultancy Services at Mumbai, Maharashtra, India. He is nationally renowned as one of the finest in this field. This edition, like the previous edition, has been greatly enriched by this master contribution from him. I am indeed greatly obliged to him for his kind gesture.

My wife, Dr Meera Desai, my daughter, Ushma, my son, Shlok, my daughter-in-law-to-be Prathana; and Dr Purvi Patel, my associate in many of my educational undertakings, need special thanks for their great support and backing they have given me in my entire academic career, in general, and in this project, in particular.

I am grateful to Shri Jitendar P Vij (Group Chairman), Mr Ankit Vij (Group President), Ms Chetna Malhotra Vohra (Associate Director-Content Strategy), Ms Ritika Chandna (Development Editor) and others at M/s Jaypee Brothers Medical Publishers, New Delhi, India, and their staff, for their help in preparation of this book.

Last but not least, I bow down in prayer to the presiding deities of learning and wisdom *Maa Saraswati* and *Lord Ganesh* for their immeasurable blessings and approval. I place this new edition of this book at their feet with complete adoration and in total devotion.

Contents

1. **Introduction to Recurrent Spontaneous Miscarriages—An Overview**   1
   - Recurrent Spontaneous Miscarriages and Obstetric Vasculopathies   2

2. **Ultrasonographic Features of Fetal Demise**   4
   - Terminology   4
   - Gestational Sac Features   4
   - Subchorionic Hemorrhage   6
   - Fetal Cardiac Activity   9
   - Yolk Sac   14
   - Doppler Findings   16

3. **Anatomical Causes of Recurrent Spontaneous Miscarriages**   17
   - European Society of Human Reproduction and Embryology/European Society for Gynaecological Endoscopy Consensus on Diagnosis of Female Genital Anomalies   18
   - Congenital Uterine Anomalies   22
   - Acquired Uterine Anomalies   28
   - Cervical Incompetence   31

4. **Immunology of Recurrent Pregnancy Miscarriage**   42
   - Hyperhomocysteinemia and Recurrent Miscarriage   43
   - Systemic Lupus Erythematosus   44
   - Leads for Obstetric Vasculopathies through Recurrent Spontaneous Abortion   44
   - Fetus as an Allograft   44
   - Partner Specificity in Miscarriages   54
   - Autoimmunity in Recurrent Pregnancy Loss   56
   - The Miracle of Paradox   67

- Laboratory Evaluation 68
- Treatment 69

5. **Genetics of Recurrent Miscarriages and Other Pregnancy Losses** 77
   Sharad Gogate
   - Etiology 77
   - Blighted Ovum and Missed Abortion 81
   - Syndromes 84
   - Chromosomal Abnormalities and Fetal Malformations 84
   - Investigative Workup for Genetic Causes of Recurrent Pregnancy Loss 85
   - Genetic Counseling 90
   - Management 91

6. **Endocrinal Causes of Recurrent Spontaneous Miscarriages** 94
   - Diabetes and Recurrent Spontaneous Miscarriages 95
   - Thyroid Abnormalities and Recurrent Spontaneous Miscarriages 95
   - Progesterone and Recurrent Spontaneous Miscarriages 96
   - Progesterone and Human Chorionic Gonadotropins Supplementation in the Treatment of Recurrent Spontaneous Miscarriages 98
   - Luteinizing Hormone Endocrinopathy and Recurrent Spontaneous Miscarriages 103
   - Polycystic Ovarian Syndrome—Insulin Resistance and Recurrent Pregnancy Loss 106

7. **Endometriosis and Recurrent Spontaneous Miscarriages** 115
   - Endometriosis and Pregnancy Loss— Examining the Evidence 115
   - Possible Causes of Endometriosis and Pregnancy Loss 117

8. Infections and Recurrent Spontaneous Miscarriages — 121
- Essentials of Laboratory Diagnosis for Proving the Association between Specific Organism and Recurrent Pregnancy Loss *123*
- Specific Infections and Recurrent Pregnancy Loss *124*

9. Psychological Bearings of Recurrent Miscarriages — 129
- Immunology, Psychology and Recurrent Pregnancy Loss *130*
- Providing Psychological Support to Subjects with Recurrent Pregnancy Loss *131*
- Components of Support Giving that may be Helpful *132*

10. Evidence-based Practice in Recurrent Spontaneous Miscarriages — 135
- Classification of Evidence Levels *135*
- Genetic Factors *137*
- Anatomical Factors *138*
- Cervical Weakness *139*
- Endocrinal Factors *139*
- Progesterone Supplementation *140*
- Human Chorionic Gonadotropin Supplementation *140*
- Immune Factors *141*
- Infections and Recurrent Spontaneous Abortion *142*
- Other Treatments *143*
- Allied Aspects *144*

11. Approach to a Subject with Recurrent Spontaneous Miscarriages — 148
- The First Consultation *148*
- On Conception *152*

Index — 155

Chapter 1

Introduction to Recurrent Spontaneous Miscarriages—An Overview

INTRODUCTION

In any living organism, reproductive system is the most complex and advanced of all systems. It could probably be because the living organism is reproducing itself. In spite of the most advanced technology and remarkable developments in modern engineering, there is no machine built till date which can manufacture its kind. The reproductive system precisely does this, effortlessly. The price that it pays for this impressive capability is wastefulness. When one encounters an entire system which is inherently wasteful, the amazement knows no bounds. It is logical to wonder as to why this inefficiency? Is it the price it pays to be the most specialized system or something else we do not know? Elsewhere in nature, one sees so many flowers bloom of which there are so few fruits. So, the inefficiency of this system may not be confined only to human beings or animals but to the entire biological world. Single or anecdotal failure may be explainable by the specialization of this system. But why does it fail repeatedly? This repeated failure is what precisely this monogram tries to explore and explain.

Advances in reproductive biology occur at a fast pace. Understanding of the pheno-mena of recurrent spontaneous miscarriages also has its share of changes. The term abortion is now replaced by miscarriage. Also, words like missed abortion have been replaced by embryonic demise or fetal demise as per the duration of pregnancy at which this has occurred.

Immunology is the most important, complex, and most prevalent cause of recurrent pregnancy miscarriage. Intolerance to a foreign protein is a protective mechanism. It is the same intolerance which rejects grafts and transplanted tissue and organs. This robustly protective system is expected to make an exception for the conceptus. The mother, who rejects every organ and tissue donated by the father, not only tolerates but protects and nourishes his conceptus. This phenomenon is no short of a miracle. Failure of this protective system leads to graft rejection and in this case, causes a miscarriage. Rejection can occur repeatedly and cause a recurrent spontaneous miscarriage. Circulating antibodies also cause the graft to "runt" and undergo a failure to thrive. Therefore, immunology seems to be the most important cause of recurrent spontaneous miscarriages in clinical practice.

RECURRENT SPONTANEOUS MISCARRIAGES AND OBSTETRIC VASCULOPATHIES

Currently, the concept of obstetric vasculopathies has also become very popular. In simplest terms, obstetric vasculopathy means disease of vessels resulting from an obstetric event. All those clinical conditions which have a placental vascular origin are grouped as obstetric vasculopathies. Interestingly, all of them have a common immunological basis. Obstetric vasculopathies include:
- Recurrent spontaneous missed miscarriages of late 1st trimesters and 2nd trimesters.
- Accidental hemorrhage with association of intrauterine growth restriction (IUGR) or preeclampsia.
- A fetal demise in a nonanomalous pregnancy with an association of any one of the earlier conditions.

Endocrinal causes that cause recurrent spontaneous miscarriages have many aspects hidden and some revealed. The role of insulin resistance and high luteinizing hormone (LH) has come into focus over a period of time. It is perceived that these cause infertility as well as recurrent spontaneous miscarriages. This aspect has been reviewed in details in the pages to follow.

Infertility and miscarriages are two medical conditions which have a profound effect on the couple as well as the entire family. In societies like India where even a routine obstetric antenatal sonography becomes a social event, miscarriage is bound to have its effects beyond the couple. Often in clinical practice does one encounter couples who are exasperated and frustrated by their repeatedly failing reproductive system and they need psychiatric support.

Anatomical defects in the uterus, both congenital and acquired can profoundly alter the uterine milieu. Conceptus in such an altered milieu can cause recurrent pregnancy failure. Sometimes, altered uterine milieu may not be as hostile to the conceptus as can be the cervical inefficiency. Cervical incompetence as it is more popularly referred to may be innate to the cervix itself or secondary to the altered uterine milieu. Its management can be very challenging to handle.

With the recent advances in assisted reproductive technology, recurrent implantation failure is one more aspect of recurrent spontaneous miscarriages that has come into focus. It needs to be carefully understood and its management scientifically handled.

Gray areas in recurrent miscarriages are many. These include endometriosis, some endocrinopathy, and psychological basis of recurrent miscarriages. However, none of the infections have been proved to cause recurrent spontaneous miscarriages. In the following chapters of this monogram, all these aspects have been extensively reviewed and explained.

Chapter 2

Ultrasonographic Features of Fetal Demise

INTRODUCTION

An ultrasound performed during the 1st trimester is crucial in diagnosing early pregnancy failure and ectopic pregnancy. As sonographic spatial resolution improved 1st trimester sonography increasingly also offers early pregnancy screening for chromosomal abnormalities and fetal structural abnormalities. The fundamental requirement for any obstetrician who intends to handle subjects with recurrent spontaneous miscarriages is to know how to diagnose a miscarriage on ultrasonography (USG). This chapter has therefore been included in this monogram on recurrent spontaneous miscarriages.

TERMINOLOGY

A commonly used term missed abortion seems to be hiding more than it reveals. It will, therefore, be scientific to use some more specific terminology. The term embryonic demise is advocated when there is evidence on a nonliving embryo. The term blighted ovum should be used in situations when there is a clear evidence of an abnormal pregnancy with a gestational sac (GS) but no visible embryo. Simplifying, therefore, it would be prudent to describe an abnormal intrauterine pregnancy as unsuccessful or failed pregnancy.

GESTATIONAL SAC FEATURES

An early normal intrauterine GS often can transabdominally be identified by 31-days gestational age (GA) and can consistently be identified by 35-days GA. To confidently diagnose an intrauterine pregnancy most observers rely on the double decidual sac finding, which is not universally present until the mean sac diameter is 10 mm corresponding to 40 days of GA. In normal gestation, mean sac growth is 1.13 mm/day; in comparison, mean sac growth in an abnormal intrauterine pregnancy is 0.70 mm/day. Based on these observations, abnormal sac growth can be diagnosed confidently if the GS fails to grow by at least 0.6 mm/day indicating a possible fetal demise.

An empty GS of more than 16 mm diameter by transabdominal sonography (TAS) or more than 8 mm diameter by transvaginal sonography (TVS) can be alarming and can alert the obstetrician as one of the first features of pregnancy failure. Undoubtedly, a wrong menstrual date can also give a false impression of an absent embryonic shadow. However, when no such subjective disparity exists, failure to visualize an embryonic shadow at or beyond 6 weeks of pregnancy on a transvaginal ultrasound is ominous. Such an anembryonic pregnancy can show a GS which is still regular, and if this is very early embryonic demise, it may even correspond with the weeks of gestation. GS can be misleading in situations when the subject insists on a review after a week, and the obstetrician may find that the sac has increased in size. This increase is never by the weeks of gestation (always less). On subsequent visit failing to visualize the embryonic shadow again should make the obstetrician confident of an embryonic demise.

It is true that GS measurements may not be very helpful in monitoring a pregnancy once crown-rump length (CRL) is measurable. Also, it is recommended that GS should be determined by measuring the mean sac diameter (MSD). It is obtained by adding the three orthogonal dimensions of the chorionic cavity (excluding the surrounding echogenic rim of tissue) and dividing by three.[1] However, GS does develop distinctive features on a failing or a failed pregnancy. The irregularity of a GS is one feature which has long been described as suggestive of a failed pregnancy. Also dismal is the failure of the sac to grow uniformly in all directions. A GS to CRL disparity can warn of a possible demise. From 5.5 weeks to 9 weeks GA, the mean GS size is usually at least 5 mm greater than the CRL.

When this difference is less than 5 mm, the subsequent spontaneous miscarriage rate exceeds 90%. The cause for this 1st trimester oligohydramnios is uncertain, but this observation suggests that with suboptimal 1st trimester GS enlargement, a high likelihood of pregnancy loss exists. At the same time, a slow rate of growth in CRL is also indicative of a possible fetal demise.

SUBCHORIONIC HEMORRHAGE

Overhyped and hardly of much clinical significance presence of a large area of subchorionic hemorrhage (SCH) was thought to be predictive of a fetal demise. It results from abruption of placental margin or a marginal sinus rupture. It is often remote from the placenta. Acute SCH is usually hyperechoic or isoechoic in relation to the placenta. It becomes sonolucent in 1-2 weeks. Identification of SCH is associated with 60-70% continuation rate when with a positive cardiac activity (CA). It is a common perception that if SCH is more than 50% of the size of chorionic tissue fetal demise is imminent. However, this too may not be a universal rule. There are reports wherein pregnancies with SCH larger than 50% have had successful outcomes.

If one is interested in the pathogenesis of SCH, it would not be difficult to understand as to why SCH is not a good predictor of pregnancy continuance or otherwise. It is now very well proved that the rejection or acceptance of a fetal allograft depends to a large extent on cytokines. Broadly speaking there are two types of cytokines—(1) The protective cytokines, and (2) The destructive cytokines. It was previously believed that these cytokines mediate through chorionic cells. If the protective cytokines supervene (which is the usual case), pregnancy continues unhindered. However, if the destructive cytokines overwhelm their protective brethren, the outcome is unsurprisingly a failure of gestation.

It has recently been proved that cytokines do not act or through the cells but through the vascular channels. Thus, the struggle between the protective and destructive cytokines occurs in the vascular bed. The presence of an area of SCH, therefore, is simply indicative of this "war." It is a marker of the fact that "the tussle" is on leading to disruption of vessel walls. It no way can predict the outcome. Thus, the presence of an area of SCH only indicates the ongoing tussle. It should not be given undue importance or be given an edificial position of a sensitive predictor of pregnancy outcome.

There is a conventional wisdom which suggests that if the area covered by SCH is more than 50% of the chorionic plate than the prognosis is poor. However, what is more important is to correlate the presence of SCH with fetal growth and CA. If the growth is corresponding with the weeks of gestation and CA is present, then the prognosis is not bad.

Case Study 1

Mrs MA presented to us with history of three pregnancy failures. This time she had pregnancy of 7 weeks with spotting P/V. Her USG picture is shown in Figure 2.1. It is interesting to note that the area of SCH was quite large. It resembled a fibroid uterus. However, on a better USG, it was clear that this was SCH. However, the fetus was corresponding with the weeks of gestation, and CA was normal. Soon the bleeding stopped, and the pregnancy thrived.

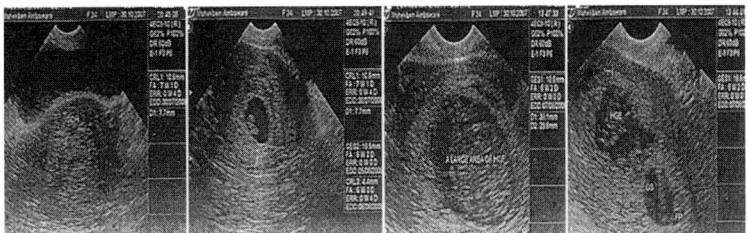

Fig. 2.1: Mrs MA: Large area of SCH at 7 weeks of pregnancy.

Her 32-weeks scan showed normal liquor amnii as shown in Figure 2.2. Vascular flows through critical vessels of the fetus were also normal. Flow through middle cerebral artery (MCA) flow is shown in Figure 2.3. The pregnancy continued uneventfully. Her cardiotocography (CTG) picture at 36 weeks is shown in Figure 2.4.

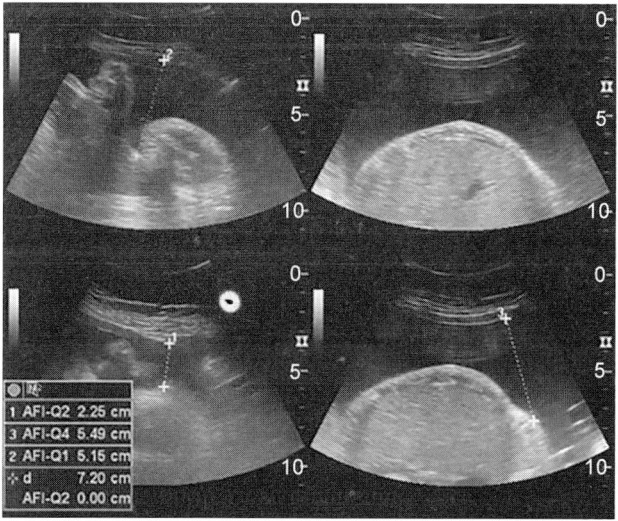

Fig. 2.2: Mrs MA: Liquor amnii at 32 weeks. (AFI: amniotic fluid index)

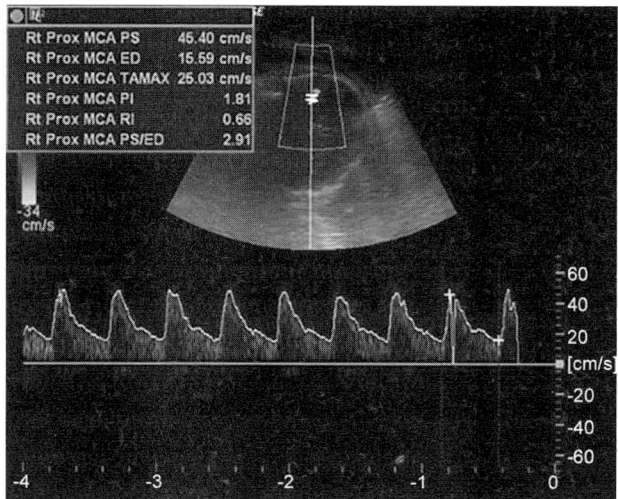

Fig. 2.3: Mrs MA: Middle cerebral artery (MCA) flow at 32 weeks.

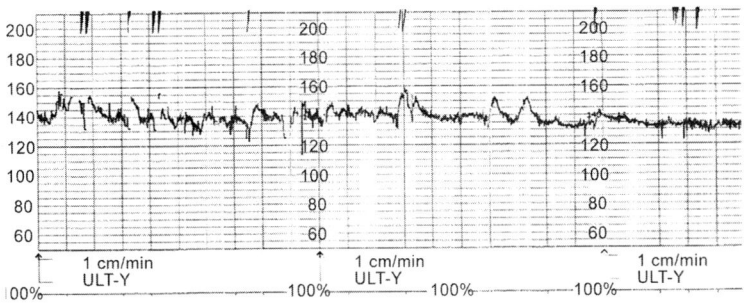

Fig. 2.4: Mrs MA: Cardiotocography (CTG) picture at 36 weeks.

Result

She delivered a full-term live baby of 3.4 kg in weight by lower segment cesarean section (LSCS). LSCS was done for cephalopelvic disproportion (CPD).

FETAL CARDIAC ACTIVITY

A very sensitive and specific parameter to conclude a fetal demise, it is undoubtedly the most relied upon. No doubt TVS can depict the presence of CA much earlier than the TAS, however, failure to demonstrate CA in an embryo or a fetus which may still be corresponding with the weeks of gestation nearly gives away the diagnosis of fetal demise.

When using a transabdominal approach, 9 mm should be considered the discriminatory CRL for detecting CA. Utilized in this manner, the discriminatory level denotes the numeric value when a certain finding should always be present. Given its superior resolution, vaginal ultrasound scans can detect CA with a smaller embryonic CRL. When a transvaginal approach is used, 4 mm is considered the discriminatory embryonic length for detecting cardiac motion. Even 5 mm has been suggested as discriminatory embryonic size for detecting cardiac motion.[2] If an embryo exceeds the discriminatory length and CA is absent, a nonviable gestation should be diagnosed. This observation should be made by two independent observers, and interpretive caution must be exercised in any questionable case. Sonographic features of embryonic demise are shown in Box 2.1.

Box 2.1: Radiographic assessment of embryonic demise.

Major criteria
A pregnancy is considered nonviable on transvaginal ultrasound if:
- No fetal heart beat where:
  – CRL ≥ 7 mm
- No fetal pole where:
  – MSD > 25 mm with no embryo
  – If a fetal pole is present, fetal pole measurements override MSD measurement.

Both fetus and gestational sac are expected to grow 1 mm/day. Hence, absence or inadequate growth on serial scans at least 7–10 days apart is suggestive of nonviability.

Other poor prognostic indicators
No yolk sac, where:
- MSD > 8 mm
- Embryo seen
- Irregular gestational sac
- Low position of the gestational sac.

If there is an absence of heart beat in a fetus that is less than 7 mm, the diagnosis of miscarriage cannot be made with certainty. This scenario is termed "pregnancy of uncertain viability (PUV)", and follow-up with ultrasound (generally in 7–10 days) and serial βhCG recommended.

(βhCG: beta human chorionic gonadotropin; CRL: crown-rump length; MSD: mean sac diameter)

It progressively increases from 110 beats per minute at 5.5 weeks (CRL 3–4 mm) to 171–178 beats per minute at 8 weeks (CRL 15 mm). At 9 weeks the embryonic heart rate reaches a plateau ranging from 160 beats per minute to 190 beats per minute. It continues in this range into the 2nd trimester slowing then to 120–160 beats per minute.

Embryonic bradycardia is considered as a sign of impending fetal loss. Embryonic heart rate (EHR) less than 85 beats per minute (+ 2SD) was taken to be a sign of impending fetal loss.[3] The sensitivity of abnormal EHR in predicting fetal loss is 65%. Normal EHR predicted a healthy outcome in 98% subjects. Rapid EHR has two possible explanations: (1) Embryo being smaller than it should be reflecting its reduced growth capacity, and (2) EHR more than 200 beats per minute may indicate an infection. In an immunological cause of recurrent spontaneous miscarriages, the characteristic feature is a cessation of CA after it was seen at least once. A clinician should think of an immunological cause if such an element is recorded or found.

The fetal heart rate at different weeks of gestation is tabulated in Table 2.1. A remarkably slow heart rate can indicate an impending fetal demise. However, this may not be a very reliable feature; clinicians can go on-guard if they find a distinctly slow heart rate to those weeks of gestation. Though the detection of fetal heart activity confirms the presence of fetal life, if body movements are observed, detection of CA is not needed to confirm viability.

Table 2.1: Gestational age (weeks) mean fetal heart rate (beats per minute + 1 SD).

5–5.95	101.2 ± 8.7
6–6.95	124.5 ± 12.1
7–7.95	128.0 ± 11.7
8–8.95	144.3 ± 19.5
9–9.95	138.7 ± 12.4
10–10.95	136.9 ± 10.9
11–11.95	139.8 ± 18.0
12–12.95	137.3 ± 12.9

Source: Adapted from Hertzberg BS, Mahony BS, Bowie JD. First trimester fetal cardiac activity. Sonographic documentation of a progressive early rise in heart rate. J Ultrasound Med. 1988;7(10):573-5.

Case Study 2

Mrs AS had an obstetric vasculopathy in her first pregnancy. In the initial period that pregnancy proceeded uneventfully as shown in Figures 2.5 and 2.6.

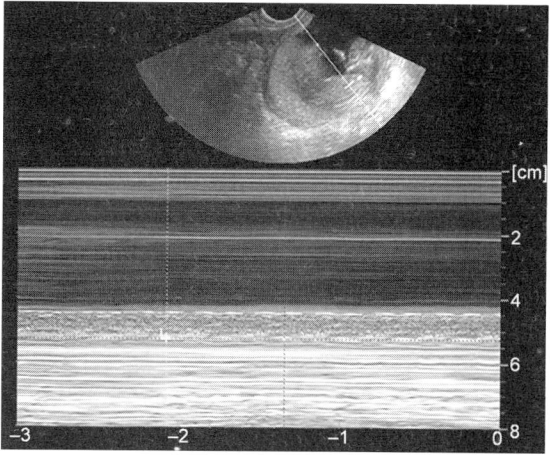

Fig. 2.5: Mrs AS: Pregnancy 1—Normal CA at 12 weeks. (CA: cardiac activity)

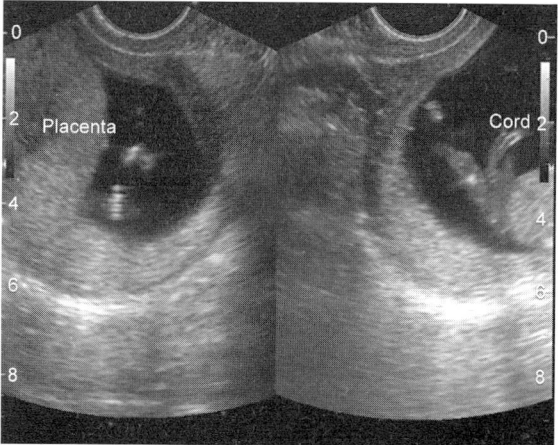

Fig. 2.6: Mrs AS: Pregnancy 1—Normal placenta and cord.

However, in the second half of pregnancy, she had pregnancy-induced hypertension (PIH) with intrauterine growth restriction (IUGR). She delivered a preterm IUGR baby of 1,500 grams which survived and is currently developing normally.

She had her second pregnancy after 4 years. Having had a history of obstetric vasculopathy, she was put on high-risk pregnancy list and was called for a USG at 8 weeks instead of the low-risk subjects in whom we do USG at 11–13 weeks. She was found to have a pregnancy of about 6 weeks size as shown, the GS was found to be irregular, and there was absent embryonic heart activity suggesting an embryonic demise as shown in Figures 2.7 to 2.9. There was SCH as shown in Figure 2.10 but she did not have any spotting per vaginum.

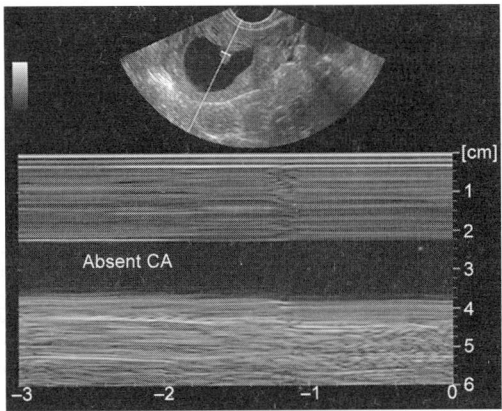

Fig. 2.7: Mrs AS: Pregnancy 2—Absent cardiac activity (CA) at 8 weeks.

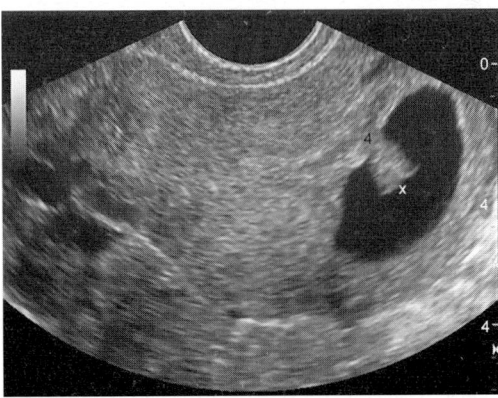

Fig. 2.8: Mrs AS: Pregnancy 2—Crown-rump length (CRL) corresponding to 6 weeks at 8 weeks gestational age.

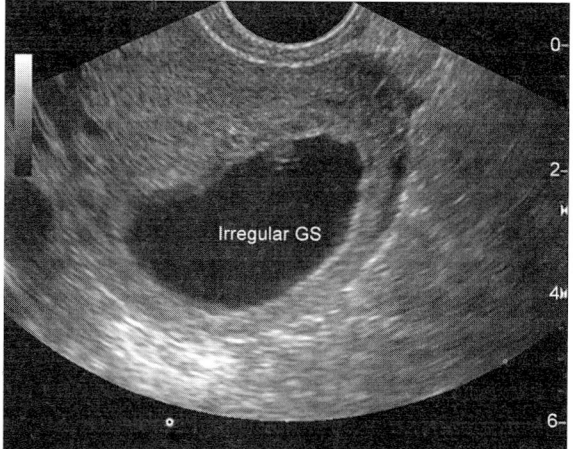

Fig. 2.9: Mrs AS: Pregnancy 2—Irregular gestational sac at 8 weeks.

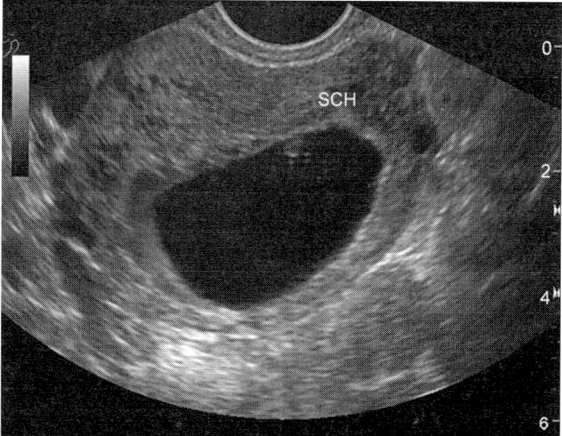

Fig. 2.10: Mrs AS: Pregnancy 2—Diffuse areas of subchorionic hemorrhage (SCH) at 8 weeks gestational age.

YOLK SAC

The yolk sac forms by 28 menstrual days and is the first structure visible in the GS. Usually, it should be seen on a transabdominal scan when the MSD is 20 mm or larger. This picture corresponds to a GA of 7 weeks. Transvaginal transducers can uniformly detect the yolk sac when the MSD is 8 mm or larger 12 mm. It corresponds to a GA of 5.5 weeks. Failure to visualize a yolk sac when the GA has reached these discriminatory values signals the pregnancy is not progressing normally.

While not much significance is attributed to yolk sac assessment, there are indeed some features which when looked at comprehensively with other parameters can reinforce the diagnosis of a fetal demise. An abnormal appearing yolk sac also can predict subsequent death. Abnormal features include large size (diameter greater than 6 mm), calcification or echogenic material within the yolk sac, and a double appearance to the yolk sac (Fig. 2.11). A large yolk sac (>5–7 mm diameter) or a small yolk sac (<2 mm diameter) is ominous. Also, an irregular or enfolded yolk sac reflects sac collapse and therefore a presumptive evidence of an embryonic death. A free-floating yolk sac is also ominous and so is calcification of yolk sac as both indicate an embryonic demise. These signs often proceed the fall in human chorionic gonadotropin (hCG) levels.

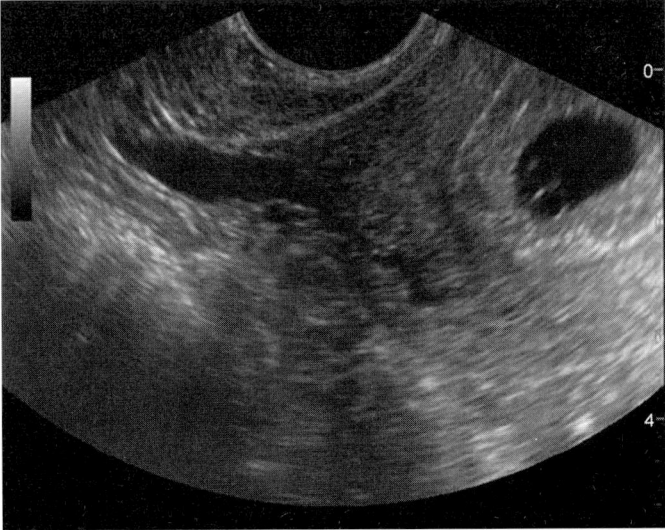

Fig. 2.11: Double yolk sac.

DOPPLER FINDINGS

Some reports suggest if the resistive index is measured at the subchorionic level and exceeds 0.55, a high likelihood of spontaneous miscarriage exists; however, others claim that Doppler analyses of these vessels are not predictive of outcome. Some qualitative observations in Doppler have been tabulated in Table 2.2.

Table 2.2: Qualitative observations on Doppler in early pregnancy loss.

Abnormal pregnancy	Trophoblastic flow	Corpus luteum (CL) flow
Embryonic demise	Poor or absent	Normal
Anembryonic pregnancy	Normal	Normal
Deficient CL	Normal	Poor or absent
Chromosomal	Normal	Normal

REFERENCES

1. Peter C. Ultrasound Evaluation during the First Trimester of Pregnancy: Ultrasonography in Obstetrics and Gynecology, 5th edition. New Delhi: Elsevier; 2008.
2. Pennell RG, Needleman L, Pajak T, et al. Prospective comparison of vaginal and abdominal sonography in normal early pregnancy. J Ultrasound Med. 1991;10(2):63-7.
3. Laboda LA, Estroff JA, Benacerraf BR. First trimester bradycardia. A sign of impending fetal loss. J Ultrasound Med. 1989;8(10):561-3.

Chapter 3

Anatomical Causes of Recurrent Spontaneous Miscarriages

INTRODUCTION

Abnormalities of the uterus are relatively common and might make embryo implantation and fetal development difficult. It may lead to infertility, pregnancy loss, preterm labor and delivery, and malpresentations. Also, these abnormalities can produce dyspareunia and menstrual symptoms like dysmenorrhea and rarely amenorrhea. These abnormalities are of varied etiology and have differing and distinct clinical significance.

Congenital uterine anomalies include Müllerian abnormalities and those following maternal diethylstilbestrol (DES) exposure (Fig. 3.1). Acquired abnormalities that can develop during a woman's lifetime include benign uterine lesions like leiomyomas and polyps and uterine scarring from diverse causes. Impaired vascularization and fetal growth restriction due to uterine distortion are the commonly considered reasons for pregnancy loss in such women. Many of these anomalies are amenable to surgical correction; hence, early and accurate diagnosis helps in optimizing reproductive performance.

The presence of a uterine anomaly might not always result in pregnancy loss, and many women with such anomalies do have healthy pregnancy outcomes. In a comparative study, the relative incidence of uterine anomalies was similar in women with and without a history of recurrent miscarriage.[1] The difference in pregnancy outcomes is explainable by the fact that distortion of uterine anatomy was more severe in women with a history of recurrent 1st trimester miscarriage. It should also be understood that

Recurrent Spontaneous Miscarriages

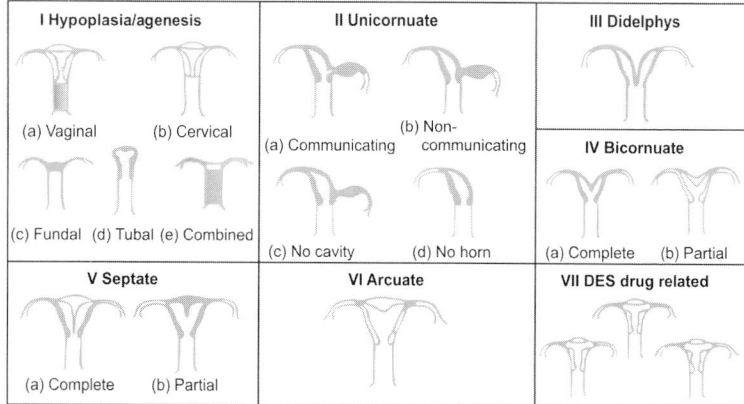

Fig. 3.1: Classification of uterine anomalies. (DES: diethylstilbestrol)

pregnancy loss might occur in a woman with a uterine anomaly due to an entirely unrelated cause like a fetal chromosomal abnormality.

The third category includes pregnancies lost due to a weakness of the cervix, which too can be treated by surgical methods. This chapter reviews these conditions and their association with recurrent pregnancy losses and discusses current diagnosis and treatment options.

EUROPEAN SOCIETY OF HUMAN REPRODUCTION AND EMBRYOLOGY/ EUROPEAN SOCIETY FOR GYNAECOLOGICAL ENDOSCOPY CONSENSUS ON DIAGNOSIS OF FEMALE GENITAL ANOMALIES[2]

Diagnostic Methods

- *Clinical examination:* It is the essential starting point of the evaluation. It also offers unique evaluation of vaginal and cervical abnormalities.
- *Hysterosalpingography:* It provides reliable information regarding uterine anatomy in the absence of cervical obstruction. It, however, does not provide any information relating to the anatomy of the vagina. It cannot be used for diagnosing

obstructive abnormalities. Its efficacy is limited by false positive and false negatives.
- *Two-dimensional ultrasonography:* It is a reliable, objective, and measurable tool. It is an essential part of the assessment. However, it is dynamic, depends on the experience of the clinician. It needs a systematic approach.
- *Recommendations for proper use of two-dimensional ultrasonography:* The endometrial line should always be visible for precise imaging of the uterus. Serial sagittal and transverse scan should be taken extending beyond the margins of the uterus.
- *Hysterosalpingo-contrast sonography:* Early follicular phase is recommended to avoid pregnancy and artifacts due to thick secretory endometrium.
- *Three-dimensional ultrasonography:* It can provide highly reliable, objective, and most importantly, measurable information for the anatomy of the female genital tract. This information includes the anatomy of the cervix, uterine cavity, uterine wall, and the external contour of the uterus. It can also provide information for associated pelvic pathology. The coronal plane imaging of the uterus provides a clear image of the cavity and the external profile of the uterine fundus. Three-dimensional (3D) volumes give a reliable and objective representation of the examined organs more independently of the examiner overcoming the limitations of obtaining coronal images with two-dimensional (2D) sonography. It can provide, also, measurable information even for obstructed parts of the female genital tract.
- *Recommendations for proper use of three-dimensional ultrasonography:* This method should be started with a 2D evaluation of the uterus. Use in midcycle or luteal phase is encouraged as this demonstrates the endometrial wall and the outline of the cavity at its best. Contrast medium could be utilized for the evaluation of the cavity and the tubes; in these cases, the examination has to be performed in the early follicular phase. Save a 3D volume for off-line analysis. The reconstructed coronal plane of the uterus might show the cavity and the external uterine profile as well as the tubal angle and the junctional zone,

if possible along all the endometrium and cavity. Diagnosis of associated vaginal anomalies can be done by a transperineal acquisition of the pelvic floor volume after filling the vagina with gel or saline; an axial plane can be obtained from a midsagittal plane.

- *Magnetic resonance imaging:* It is noninvasive, and it has no radiation. It gives a reliable and objective representation of the examining organs in the sagittal, transverse, and coronal plane (three dimensions). It can be used for diagnosis in cases of complex and obstructing anomalies. Electronic storage of the diagnostic procedure is, nowadays, routinely done for re-evaluation.
- *Hysteroscopy:* It is minimally invasive giving the additional opportunity of treating T-shaped, septate, and bicorporeal septate uterus. Its objective includes estimation of the cervical canal and endometrial cavity (differential diagnosis of a T-shaped and infantile uterus). Electronic storage of the procedure is, nowadays, routinely done for re-evaluation.
- *Endoscopy:* Laparoscopy and hysteroscopy provide highly reliable information for the anatomical status of the vagina (vaginoscopic approach), cervical canal, uterine cavity, tubal ostia, external contour of the uterus, and the intraperitoneal structures.
- The invasiveness of the laparoscopic approach makes it not acceptable as a first-line screening procedure; it complements indirect imaging in the diagnosis of more complex anomalies in combination with possible surgical actions. It offers supplementary information about the partial or total absence of fallopian tubes and abnormal localization of ovaries.
- Highest degrees of overall diagnostic accuracy were in decreasing order: 3D ultrasound (US) (97.6%), sonohysterography (SHG; 96.5%), 2D US (86.6), and hysterosalpingography (HSG; 86.9%). Magnetic resonance imaging (MRI) was shown to subclassify 85.8% of anomalies correctly. Overall, it appears that 3D US may be more accurate than MRI in subclassifying malformations, although it should be noted that subclassification is hindered due to the subjective nature of the previous classifications adopted.

Uterine Wall Thickness

- Uterine wall thickness is an important parameter and a reference point for the definitions of dysmorphic T-shaped, septate, and bicorporeal uteri according to the new classification system. The adoption of an objective criterion for the definition of uterine deformity is one of the advantages of the new classification system, since according to American Fertility Society (AFS) classification the detection of anomalies was based only on the subjective impression of the clinician performing the test. Although myometrial thickness at the various uterine regions cannot be easily assessed with endoscopic techniques, it can be measured with US or MRI.
- Uterine wall thickness is the distance between the line connecting the tubal ostia and the external uterine profile obtained with 3D US, MRI, and at times, with 2D ultrasonography (USG).

Although US can only identify about half of the congenital uterine anomalies present, its diagnosis is very likely to be correct due to its meager false-positive rate. Therefore, it could prove to be a handy screening tool in conjunction with HSG since they are both widely available. HSG does not evaluate the external contour of the uterus, and therefore it cannot reliably differentiate between a septate and a bicornuate uterus. It provides valuable information regarding the interior cavity of the uterus. When it shows a unicornuate uterus, a second cervical opening must be looked for and if found further injection of contrast into the cervix may lead to the diagnosis of a uterine didelphys or a complete septate uterus. In assessing a unicornuate uterus with HSG, blocked or noncommunicating rudimentary horns will not appear on film. Using a saline contrast during transvaginal US examination (saline infusion SHG or SIS) gives better results than either US or HSG alone. Reports comparing SIS with hysteroscopy have suggested that SIS is highly accurate in both diagnosing and categorizing congenital uterine anomalies.[3]

Three-dimensional US and MRI have the advantage of being more accurate and noninvasive in the diagnosis of congenital uterine anomalies but are available in a few centers only. 3D US is a noninvasive method of investigation. It works by attaining an initial 2D US image of the uterus and storing it on to a computer. A vaginal transducer then performs a sweep of transversal sections which are also subsequently stored. The computer then integrates the images and allows the investigator to view images of three planes simultaneously. This 3D image, along with the complete volume scan, can be stored for later viewing and appraisal. Reports suggest that 3D US has a very high accuracy rate in diagnosing congenital uterine anomalies, although further studies are required to confirm this.

The gold standard of diagnosis is by a combination of hysteroscopy and laparoscopy.[4] Hysteroscopy allows the diagnosis and simultaneous treatment of many intrauterine abnormalities. Simultaneous laparoscopy is often necessary to visualize the uterine fundus and reliably differentiate between a septate and bicornuate uterus. The main disadvantage of this technique is in it being invasive.[5]

CONGENITAL UTERINE ANOMALIES

Müllerian duct malformations delineate a miscellaneous group of congenital anomalies that result from arrested development, abnormal formation, or incomplete fusion of the mesonephric ducts (Box 3.1). Though the actual incidence is not known, various studies have suggested an incidence of 3-5% of the general population and 5-10% in women with poor reproductive outcomes.[6-8] The difference seen among various studies may be due to the population studied (fertile, infertile, or women with recurrent pregnancy loss), the method of diagnostic evaluation and whether laparohysteroscopy was used. It could also be due to inconsistent interpretation of the classification of congenital uterine anomalies. In a retrospective, longitudinal study of 3,181 patients found the overall frequency of uterine malformations of 4%. Infertile patients (6.3%) had a significantly higher incidence of Müllerian anomalies, in comparison with fertile (3.8%) and sterile (2.4%) women. It was observed that septate and arcuate uteri represented approximately 75% of the malformations, while bicornuate, didelphys, and unicornuate comprised the remaining 25%.[6] Pregnancy outcomes in women with uterine abnormalities are related to the defect in the uterine cavity and restoration of a normal cavity forms the basis of treatment.

> **Box 3.1:** Classification anomaly (American Fertility Society, 1988).[4]
>
> - *Class I*: Segmental Müllerian agenesis-hypoplasia:
>   - Vaginal
>   - Cervical
>   - Fundal
>   - Tubal
>   - Combined anomalies
> - *Class II*: Unicornuate:
>   - Communicating
>   - Noncommunicating
>   - No cavity
>   - No horn
> - *Class III*: Didelphys
> - *Class IV*: Bicornuate:
>   - Complete (complete division down to internal os)
>   - Partial
> - *Class V*: Septate:
>   - Complete (septum to internal os)
>   - Partial
> - *Class VI*: Arcuate
> - *Class VII*: Diethylstilbestrol related

Septate Uterus (Class V)

It is the most common congenital anomaly of the uterus, comprising approximately 55% of all anomalies.[9] Persistence of the uterine septum results from a lack of resorption of the midline septum between the two Müllerian ducts. Such a persistent septum may project minimally from the fundus as in an arcuate uterus or may extend downwards till the internal os to divide the endometrial cavity (Figs. 3.2 and 3.3). Rarely, a complete failure in resorption may cause a longitudinal vaginal septum.

Among the Müllerian anomalies, uterine septa are the most common cause of pregnancy loss. Fortunately, this anomaly is the easiest to treat. A reproductive loss probably occurs in the 1st trimester due to poor vascularity if the pregnancy implants on the septum. Loss latter in pregnancy in the form of midtrimester miscarriage or preterm labor may occur due to the reduced and

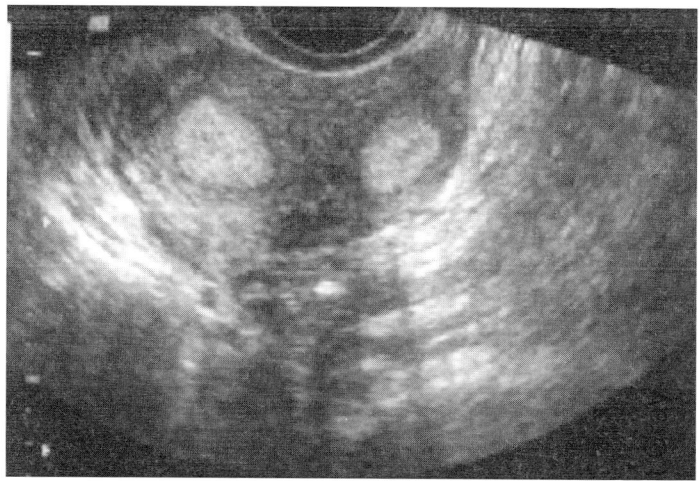

Fig. 3.2: Ultrasonography (USG) picture: Coronal section of the uterus showing two separate endometrial cavities.

distorted uterine cavity. The same reason may be the cause for fetal malpresentation.

Posttreatment reproductive outcomes are excellent with operative hysteroscopy. Although preoperative hormonal therapy causes atrophy of the endometrium and reduces vascularization and intraoperative bleeding, it also reduces the depth of the myometrium and therefore increases the risk of perforation and myometrial damage. It is suggested that surgery is performed immediately after the end of menstrual bleeding. Laparoscopy is first conducted to rule out a bicornuate uterus. It also helps in reducing the risk of perforation at the time of hysteroscopy. Incision of the septum is usually performed with a resectoscope and an electrode (Collin's knife) using pure cutting current. It can alternatively be done with hysteroscopic scissors or neodymium-doped yttrium aluminum garnet (Nd:YAG) laser. There is no role for transabdominal metroplasty for the treatment of uterine septum. The vaginal septum is excised if the woman has dyspareunia. Operative complications include perforation, hemorrhage, infection, and fluid overload. Use of postoperative hormones or insertion of an intrauterine device though practiced by some practitioners is not routinely recommended. Posttreatment miscarriage rates are approximately that of the average population.[10-12]

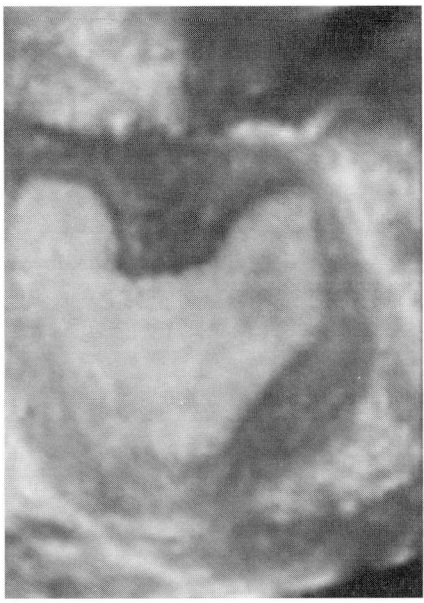

Fig. 3.3: Three-dimensional (3D) ultrasound of the same patient showing partial septum which was confirmed on laparohysteroscopy.

Bicornuate Uterus (Class IV)

This anomaly is a result of an incomplete fusion of the uterine horns at the level of the fundus. The distinguishing aspect of this anomaly is the presence of two separate but communicating endometrial cavities and a single cervix (Fig. 3.4). It represents around 10% of Müllerian duct anomalies. The degree of incomplete Müllerian fusion appears to affect the reproductive outcome. In a review of four studies comprising 261 patients with a bicornuate uterus, the mean miscarriage rate was 36%, the average preterm delivery rate was 23%, and a mean live-birth rate was 55.2%.[13] A study reported a 29% incidence of preterm delivery in women with a partial bicornuate uterus and a 66% rate of preterm delivery in women with complete bicornuate uterus.[14] Surgical correction with the Strassman metroplasty is reserved for selected patients with repeated poor pregnancy outcome.

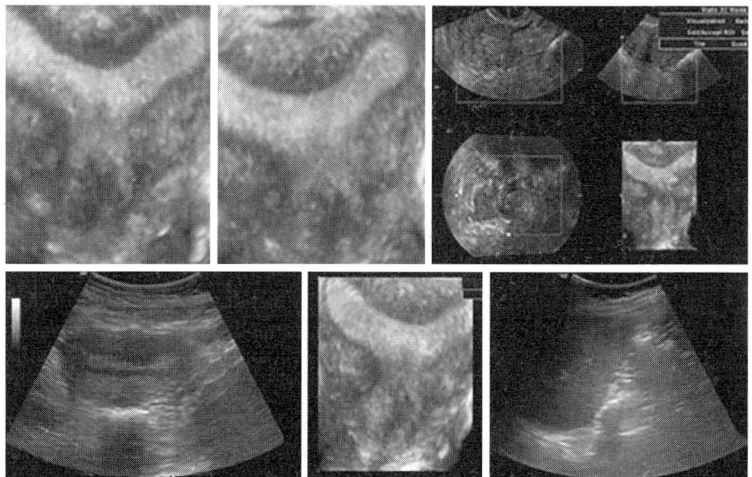

Fig. 3.4: USG picture of bicornuate uterus.
(2D: two-dimensional; 3D: three-dimensional; USG: ultrasonography)

Unicornuate Uterus (Class II)

A unicornuate uterus occurs in approximately 20% of uterine anomalies.[9] Variations of this anomaly occur due to presence or absence of the rudimentary horn (Box 3.1). Hypoplasia of one of the Müllerian ducts results in a rudimentary uterine horn, which may or may not have a cavity. Further classification is determined by whether or not the uterine horn communicates with the fully differentiated uterus. If a rudimentary horn is present with a cavity, the patient may present with unilateral cyclical pelvic pain secondary to hematometra. Associated renal anomalies, usually of the kidney occur in 40% of patients.

The altered uterine configuration is associated with an increase in obstetrical complications (miscarriages, ectopic pregnancy, malpresentations, fetal growth restriction, and preterm labor). In a review of 151 women with a unicornuate uterus, who had a total of

260 pregnancies, the mean miscarriage rate was 37.1%, the average preterm delivery rate was 16.4%, and the average live-birth rate was 55.1%.[4]

Pregnancy loss may be associated with the reduced intraluminal volume along with poor vascularity. Surgical treatment involves resection of the rudimentary horn to treat dysmenorrhea and hematometra as well as to obviate the potential for ectopic pregnancy and uterine rupture. The higher prevalence of cervical incompetence in uterine anomalies, however, has led some authors to recommend that cervical cerclage be placed to improve obstetrical outcome. Based on the currently available evidence, women with a unicornuate uterus and no previous history of 2nd trimester loss or premature birth should be managed expectantly with frequent assessment of cervical length and anatomy.[13,14]

Uterus Didelphys (Class III)

Duplication of the uterine corpus and cervix occurs due to lack of fusion of the two Müllerian ducts. Most women are asymptomatic and usually have no difficulties with menstruation and coitus. Associated renal anomalies may be present. Pregnancy is associated with an increased risk of miscarriage, malpresentations, and premature labor. In a review of 152 pregnancies by 114 patients, the mean miscarriage rate was 32.9%, the preterm delivery rate was 28.9%, and live-birth rate was 56.6%.[4] This is quite similar to the pregnancy rates seen in women with a unicornuate uterus. Surgical treatment is required in those rare cases where one side is obstructed.

Arcuate Uterus (Class VI)

Arcuate uterus might be considered as a mild form of a partial septate uterus. The near-complete resorption of the uterovaginal septum may leave a slight concave indentation of the endometrial cavity at the level of the fundus, giving the uterus an arcuate configuration. Most authors consider it to be an anatomic variant of normal with similar reproductive outcomes.[6] In a retrospective case series of 176 patients with arcuate uterus reported a 45% miscarriage rate in women.[7] Treatment is usually expectant.[8]

Diethylstilbestrol Exposure-related Anomalies (Class VII)

Diethylstilbestrol is a synthetic nonsteroidal estrogen that was used to prevent miscarriage and other pregnancy complications. Between 1938 and 1971 before the association between the development of clear cell adenocarcinoma of the vagina and cervix was found in young women whose mothers had taken DES while they were pregnant. Women who were exposed to DES in utero may have structural reproductive tract anomalies, an increased infertility rate, and poor pregnancy outcomes.[15,16] However, the majority of these women have been able to deliver successfully. The most comprehensive study to date found that 64.5% of women with in utero DES exposure had full-term infants, compared with 84.5% of matched women who had not been exposed to DES.[16] Also, the DES-exposed women had higher rates of preterm delivery (19.4% vs 7.5%), ectopic pregnancy (4.2% vs 0.77%), and 2nd trimester spontaneous miscarriage (6.3% vs 1.6%). Consequently, high-risk obstetric care may be indicated for pregnant women who were exposed to DES in utero. An incompetent cervix is common and prophylactic cerclage may be beneficial to DES-exposed women with a history of 2nd trimester loss or preterm delivery.

ACQUIRED UTERINE ANOMALIES

Benign Growths from the Myometrium and Endometrium

Uterine fibroids are often found in women of reproductive age, with 20–40% of women developing it.[17] With the current trend in delaying childbearing, there are an increasing number of women with fibroids who would come for both, treatment of infertility and antenatal care. The association between fibroids and implantation remains controversial. Some authorities believe that fibroids have a detrimental effect on implantation, either through impaired transport of gametes, altered uterine contractility, or adverse effects on the endometrium.[18] None of these hypotheses have been proven, and few have been rigorously tested.

Most authorities believe that submucous fibroids are associated with an adverse effect on implantation and placentation (Fig. 3.5). The role of intramural fibroids is controversial. Subserosal and pedunculated fibroids are unlikely to cause adverse pregnancy effects. In a review presence of submucous fibroids reduced the implantation rate from 11.5% to 3% and increased the risk of miscarriage from 22% to 47%.[18] The same authors analyzed the effects of intramural fibroids on fertility and pregnancy. This review of 19 trials on the subject showed conflicting results. A meta-analysis of these trials revealed that intramural fibroids appear to be associated with a slight decrease in implantation rate, from 22% to 18% and an increase in spontaneous miscarriage rate, from 8% to 15%. Further, well-designed studies are required in this area.

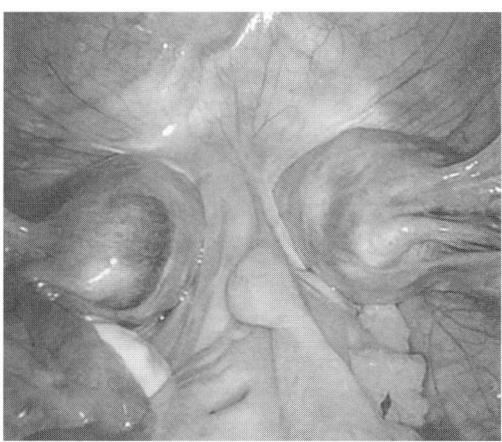

Fig. 3.5: Submucous fibroids.

Several retrospective studies have shown improvement in fertility rates after myomectomy. One study evaluated 72 patients with unexplained infertility and intramural and subserosal myomas who underwent abdominal myomectomy. The majority of subjects had one to five myomas, with sizes ranging from 3 cm to 8 cm. Statistically significant differences were found between preoperative and postoperative conception rates (28% vs 70%), live-birth rates (30% vs 75%), and miscarriage rates (69% vs 25%).[19] Hysteroscopic myomectomy is the procedure of choice in women with submucous fibroids. Relative contraindications are size more than 5 cm and more than 50% intramural extension.

Women who desire future fertility and undergo uterine artery embolization (UAE) may have lower fertility rates, and hence it is not recommended. One study compared pregnancies after UAE and laparoscopic myomectomy and found that pregnancy after UAE had a higher incidence of malpresentations and preterm labor. Spontaneous miscarriages were also similarly higher, but the difference was not statistically significant.[20]

It is thought that endometrial polyps act similar to submucous myomas in reducing fertility rates and pregnancy outcomes. It was shown that excision of polyps especially those located at the uterotubal junction significantly improved the pregnancy rates.[21] Hysteroscopic polypectomy of endometrial polyps appeared to improve fertility and increase pregnancy rates in previously infertile women with no other reason to explain their infertility, irrespective of the size or number of the polyps.[22]

Currently, medical treatments of fibroid uterus are in vogue. To what extent can medical treatment of fibroids help in treating subjects with recurrent spontaneous miscarriage still lacks good quality evidence. Recently a case report has been published that shows spontaneous pregnancy following ulipristal acetate treatment in a woman with a symptomatic uterine fibroid. Ulipristal acetate is a selective progesterone receptor modulator (SPRM). This report demonstrates the possible utility of ulipristal acetate in the management of women with symptomatic fibroids. In this report, a 35-year-old woman with a history of recurrent miscarriage (gravida 5, para 0) had a solitary submucosal fibroid extending into the uterine cavity. Following a 3-month course of ulipristal acetate 5 mg daily, fibroid volume decreased. The patient conceived approximately 2 months after discontinuing ulipristal acetate. She had an uncomplicated pregnancy and underwent a planned induction of labor at 38-weeks gestation. The patient had a normal vaginal delivery of a healthy male infant weighing 3,130 grams.[23]

Intrauterine Adhesions

Intrauterine synechia or Asherman's syndrome is an acquired uterine defect that has been associated with both infertility and recurrent pregnancy losses. The reproductive outcomes of women with Asherman's syndrome are poor. In the absence of treatment, approximately 40% of pregnancies in these women appear to end in spontaneous miscarriage, and another 23% result in preterm deliveries.[24] These adhesions are thought to decrease the volume of the uterine cavity and may interfere with the normal placentation and lead to pregnancy loss. The most common cause is instrumentation of a gravid or recently postpartum uterus. Asherman's syndrome can also result from pelvic surgeries (including cesarean sections and myomectomy), from intrauterine devices, pelvic irradiation, schistosomiasis, and genital tuberculosis. While SIS and HSG are useful as screening tests of intrauterine adhesions, hysteroscopy remains the mainstay of diagnosis and treatment. Severe intrauterine adhesions are difficult to treat, and even when a satisfying anatomical result is obtained, normal endometrial function is not guaranteed. Hysteroscopic lysis of adhesions with scissors, electrosurgery, or laser can restore the size and shape of the endometrial cavity. Significantly obliterated cavities may require multiple procedures to achieve a satisfactory anatomical result. Postoperative mechanical distention of the endometrial cavity and hormonal treatment to facilitate endometrial regrowth appear to decrease the high rate of adhesion reformation.[25] Women who conceive after treatment have a higher incidence of miscarriage. There are reports of increased incidence of uterine dehiscence and rupture and that of placenta accreta.

With the advances in assisted reproductive technology (ART) surrogacy is a viable alternative for subjects with recurrent miscarriages due to incorrigible or very severe uterine anomalies, both congenital as well as acquired.

CERVICAL INCOMPETENCE

Cervical incompetence presents with a history of recurrent second or early 3rd trimester fetal loss, after painless dilatation of the cervix, prolapse or rupture of the membranes, and expulsion of a live fetus despite minimal uterine activity.[26] Risk factors for cervical incompetence include congenital uterine anomalies, maternal DES exposure, surgeries involving the cervix, and history of trauma to the cervix. Among all uterine abnormalities, it seems bicornuate uterus is an independent risk factor for cervical os insufficiency. When found, it becomes a significant finding due to the burden of the risk for midtrimester periviable birth associated with cervical incompetence.[27]

Diagnosis is easy in women with the earlier risk factors, but in the majority of women with similar symptoms, there is a lack of uniform diagnostic criteria and an objective diagnostic test. Tests like the progressive passage of Hegar dilators (6-8 mm) through the internal cervical os, the use of balloon elastance test, or the ability of the cervix to hold an inflated Foley catheter during HSG lack evidence. Most clinicians do not wait for recurrent pregnancy loss to happen before diagnosing cervical incompetence.

A word on the role of cervical USG for diagnosis of cervical incompetence is timely. As regards the use of sonography in the antenatal diagnosis of cervical, finding of cervical funneling (Fig. 3.6), a proximal cervical length of less than 1.5 cm and a total cervical length of less than 2.5 cm have been studied. In women with a history-indicated cerclage, cervical funneling is the only independently significant sonographic finding associated with an increased risk of preterm birth before 34 weeks.[28]

In the absence of funneling, the probability of cervical incompetence is small, and the best prophylactic option is progesterone administration.[29] However, the question remains as to whether routine cervical screening by USG is justifiable for diagnosis of cervical incompetence? In one recent study, it has been shown that given the implications associated with preterm delivery, routine measurement of cervical length at the time of the anomaly scan may be justifiable from a cost point of view in a population where the risk of preterm birth is low.[30] We do a routine cervical assessment in all subjects at 11–14 weeks scan. When in doubt, one tends to seek the counsel of Cochrane database. However, in this matter as in many others, Cochrane database remains equivocal. It states that currently, there is insufficient evidence to recommend routine screening of asymptomatic or symptomatic pregnant women with measurement of cervical length by transvaginal US. Since there is a nonsignificant association between knowledge of measurement of cervical length by transvaginal US results and a lower incidence of preterm birth at less than 37 weeks in symptomatic women, they encourage further research. Future studies should look at specific populations separately (e.g. singleton versus twins, symptoms of preterm labor or no such symptoms), report on all relevant maternal and perinatal outcomes, and include cost-effectiveness analyses. Most importantly, future studies should include a clear protocol for management of women based on measurement of cervical length by transvaginal US results, so that it can be easily evaluated and replicated.[31]

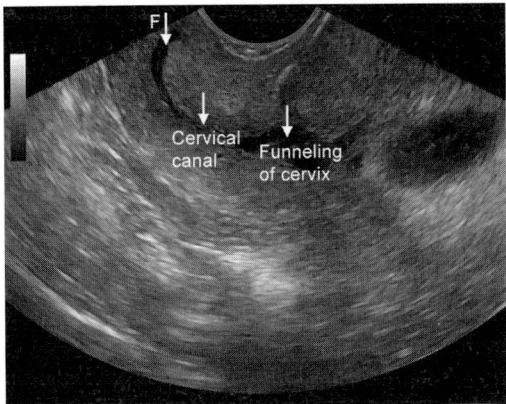

Fig. 3.6: Incompetent cervical os with funneling of proximal cervix.

In clinical practice, we routinely screen all subjects at 11–14 weeks scan for cervical length. If the cervical length is more than 3.5 cm, we do not take any steps as this is not cervical insufficiency. However, if the length is less than 2.5 cm, we examine if the subject has a history of preterm birth. If such history is forthcoming, we place a cervical cerclage stitch. In these subjects, we do not give progesterone suppository. However, in subjects with a cervical length between

2.5 cm and 3.5 cm and no history of preterm birth, we give vaginal progesterone pessaries and do not place a cervical cerclage stitch. Progesterone pessary contains natural micronized progesterone in a dose of 200 mgm twice a day. Oral micronized progesterone is also useful and is preferred in noncompliant subjects. Of late 400 mgm single dose per day and sustained release preparations are also available. Data is still limited regarding their efficacy.

Data supporting cerclage placement is limited. There has never been a prospective, randomized, and controlled trial of cerclage versus no cerclage in patients with a classic history of cervical insufficiency. Based on the current literature, there is evidence supporting cervical cerclage in the following limited circumstances:
- A history of three or more spontaneous preterm births or 2nd trimester losses.
- In a high-risk patient with a singleton pregnancy who has a short cervix in the 2nd trimester.

Because the majority of patients with risk factors for preterm birth and 2nd trimester loss will still deliver at term or near-term, studies on the effectiveness of cervical cerclage would need many patients to be powered appropriately.[32,33]

Cervical cerclage has been a common practice in obstetrics since it was first described by Shirodkar in 1955 and then by McDonald in 1957. Cerclage should be performed at 13–16 weeks of gestation after US evaluation has demonstrated the presence of a live fetus with no apparent anomalies.[34] The cerclage is removed at or about 37-weeks gestation. There are the three most important types of cerclage. The standard transvaginal cerclage is at the junction of cervix and fornix, the McDonald cerclage being the most commonly performed technique. It is essentially a purse string stitch of strong nonabsorbable material applied at the upper part of the cervix without displacing the bladder. The ends of the suture are left long to facilitate removal.

A high transvaginal cerclage is performed after opening the fornix. The Shirodkar's cerclage involves cephalad dissection and displacement of the bladder and high cerclage with a strip of fascia or synthetic tape. The third is the transabdominal cerclage at the level of the internal cervical os which can be performed by either a laparotomy or by laparoscopy. The effectiveness of these levels of cerclage has not been systematically studied. From a clinical and mechanical point of view, cervicoisthmic cerclage is superior to other cerclages as it is inserted at the level of the internal cervical os and therefore prevents funneling. From a surgical point of view, transvaginal cerclages have the advantage over transabdominal cerclage. Transvaginal surgery is shorter and easier, hospitalization is shorter, and there is no need for delivery by cesarean section. Transabdominal cerclage should probably be performed only if a transvaginal cerclage is considered technically unfeasible or hazardous because of severe cervical defects. Based on timing, various types include the prophylactic cerclage before conception, prophylactic cerclage in pregnancy, urgent cerclage after shortening of the cervix, and an emergency cerclage after dilatation of the cervix and exposure of the membranes. While performing an emergency cerclage, it might be difficult to put the stitches as mentioned earlier.

A simple closure of the external os by mattress or U-sutures might be possible (Hefner or Wurm cerclage). Emergency cerclages have traditionally been associated with a high risk of chorioamnionitis (up to 37%) and rupture of the membranes within 2 weeks of the operation (up to 65%).[25] Common complications associated with cerclage placement include cervical injury, suture displacement, rupture of membranes, and chorioamnionitis. These complications are more common when cerclage surgery is done in an emergency as compared to planned surgery.

Laparoscopic encerclage and robotic encerclage have also been performed by some workers. However, they are not better in anyway and have a limited application in clinical practice.

Case Study 1

Mrs FL presented with early pregnancy. She had been operated in another hospital for excision of vaginal septum. Papers of previous surgery were not available as she had not preserved them. On examination, she was found to have a complete didelphic uterus. Her USG picture is shown in Figure 3.7. Her clinical examination picture is shown in Figure 3.8. She continued with her pregnancy uneventfully and went on to deliver a 36-week-old 2,600 gm baby who subsequently thrived. She then after went on to conceive spontaneously and delivered one more live baby by lower segment cesarean section (LSCS) (Fig. 3.9). This case study highlights the fact that complete uterus didelphys may have a nearly uneventful outcome as in any other subject.

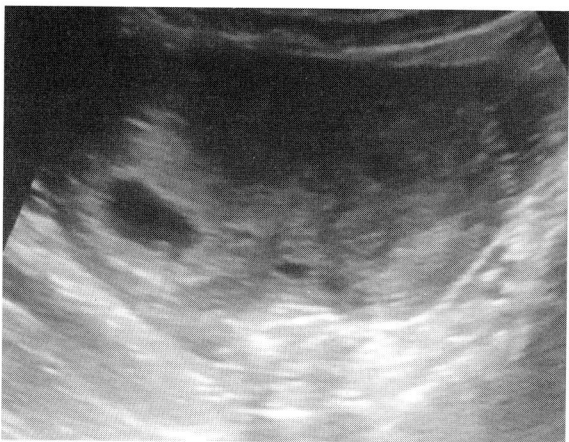

Fig. 3.7: Ultrasonography (USG) picture of uterus didelphys. Left uterus has pregnancy and right uterus is not pregnant.

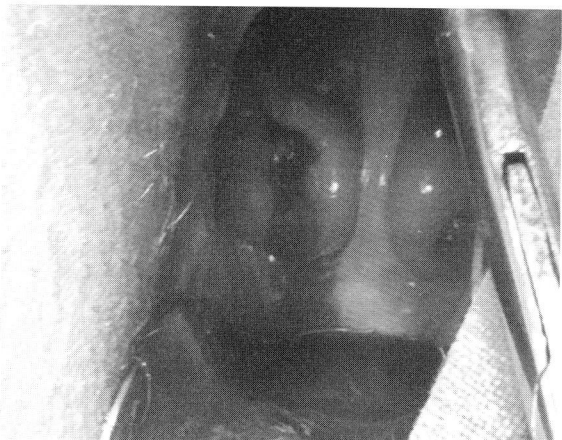

Fig. 3.8: Two well-formed cervices as seen on per-speculum examination.

Anatomical Causes of Recurrent Spontaneous Miscarriages

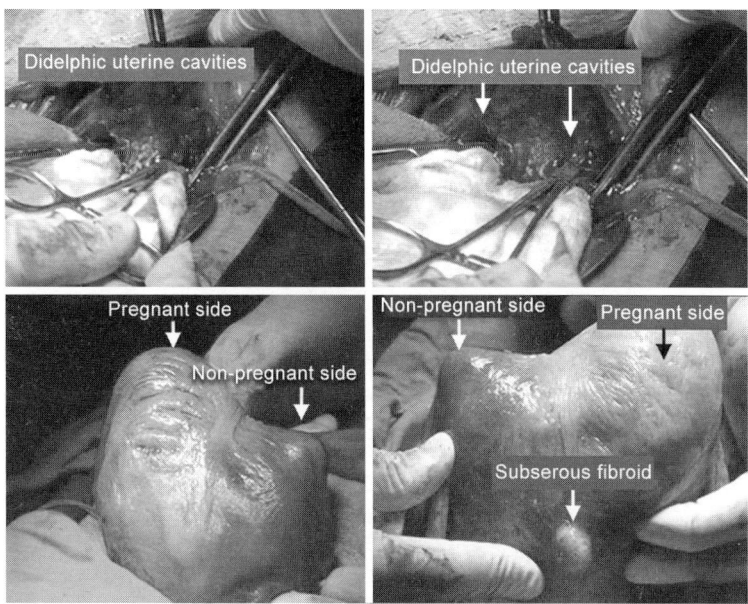

Intraoperative (LSCS) view of didelphic uterus

Fig. 3.9: Intraoperative [lower segment cesarean section (LSCS)] picture.

Case Study 2

Mrs JS presented with history of inability to conceive for last 3 years. However, while being investigated for infertility, she was found to have a bicornuate uterus. She had a spontaneous conception. At 6 weeks, her USG picture is shown in Figure 3.10. Her USG picture at 11 weeks 6 days is as shown in Figure 3.11. She was subjected to cervical cerclage prophylactically. Her pregnancy continued until 30 weeks when she had a spontaneous premature rupture of membranes and preterm labor. Baby presented by breech. Given a bicornuate uterus and primi with a breech presentation, she was subjected to LSCS. Her intraoperative pictures are as shown in Figure 3.12. The baby was a live preterm child of 1,200 gm. It was shifted to neonatal intensive care unit (NICU) and subsequently thrived. The mother had an uneventful postoperative recovery.

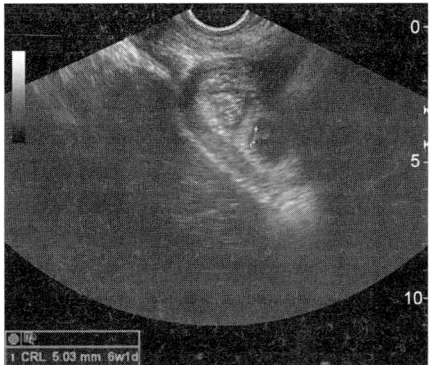

Fig. 3.10: Mrs JS: 6 weeks 1 day pregnancy in bicornuate uterus.
(CRL: crown-rump length)

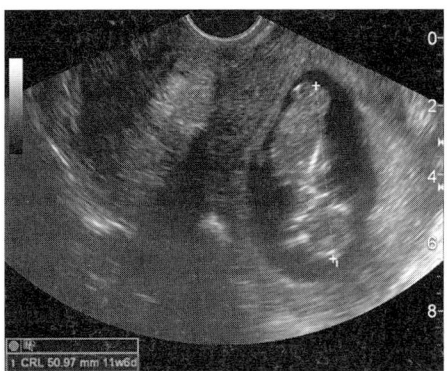

Fig. 3.11: Mrs JS: 11 weeks 6 days pregnancy in bicornuate uterus.
(CRL: crown-rump length)

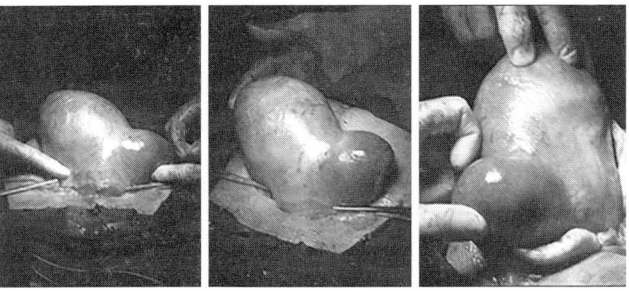

Fig. 3.12: Mrs JS: Intraoperative
[lower segment cesarean section (LSCS)] appearance of uterus.

REFERENCES

1. Salim R, Regan L, Woelfer B, et al. A comparative study of the morphology of congenital uterine anomalies in women with and without a history of recurrent first trimester miscarriage. Hum Reprod. 2003;18(1):162-6.
2. Grimbizis GF, Di Spiezio Sardo A, Saravelos SH, et al. The Thessaloniki ESHRE/ESGE consensus on diagnosis of female genital anomalies. Gynecol Surg. 2016;13:1-16.
3. Devi Wold AS, Pham N, Arici A. Anatomic factors in recurrent pregnancy loss. Semin Reprod Med. 2006;24(1):25-32.
4. Grimbizis GF, Camus M, Tarlatzis BC, et al. Clinical implications of uterine malformations and hysteroscopic treatment results. Hum Reprod Update. 2001;7(2):161-74.
5. The American Fertility Society classifications of adnexal adhesions, distal tubal occlusion, tubal occlusion secondary to tubal ligation, tubal pregnancies, müllerian anomalies and intrauterine adhesions. Fertil Steril. 1988;49(6):944-55.
6. Raga F, Bauset C, Remohi J, et al. Reproductive impact of congenital Müllerian anomalies. Hum Reprod. 1997;12(10):2277-81.
7. Acién P. Incidence of Müllerian defects in fertile and infertile women. Hum Reprod. 1997;12(7):1372-6.
8. Acién P. Reproductive performance of women with uterine malformations. Hum Reprod. 1993;8(1): 122-6.
9. Troiano RN. Magnetic resonance imaging of mullerian duct anomalies of the uterus. Top Magn Reson Imaging. 2003;14(4):269-79.
10. Homer HA, Li TC, Cooke ID. The septate uterus: a review of management and reproductive outcome. Fertil Steril. 2000;73(1):1-14.
11. Fedele L, Arcaini L, Parazzini F, et al. Reproductive prognosis after hysteroscopic metroplasty in 102 women: life-table analysis. Fertil Steril. 1993;59(4):768-72.
12. Daly DC, Maier D, Soto-Albors C. Hysteroscopic metroplasty: six years' experience. Obstet Gynecol. 1989;73(2):201-5.
13. Heinonen PK. Reproductive performance of women with uterine anomalies after abdominal or hysteroscopic metroplasty or no surgical treatment. J Am Assoc Gynecol Laparosc. 1997;4(3):311-7.
14. Abramovici H, Faktor JH, Pascal B. Congenital uterine malformations as indication for cervical suture (cerclage) in habitual abortion and premature delivery. Int J Fertil. 1983;28(3):161-4.
15. Kaufman RH, Adam E, Binder GL, et al. Upper genital tract changes and pregnancy outcome in offspring exposed in utero to diethylstilbestrol. Am J Obstet Gynecol. 1980;137(3):299-308.

16. Kaufman RH, Adam E, Hatch EE, et al. Continued follow-up of pregnancy outcomes in diethylstilbestrol-exposed offspring. Obstet Gynecol. 2000;96(4):483-9.
17. Farhi J, Ashkenazi J, Feldberg D, et al. Effect of uterine leiomyomata on the results of in-vitro fertilization treatment. Hum Reprod. 1995;10(10):2576-8.
18. Klatsky PC, Tran ND, Caughey AB, et al. Fibroids and reproductive outcomes: a systematic literature review from conception to delivery. Am J Obstet Gynecol. 2008;198(4):357-66.
19. Marchionni M, Fambrini M, Zambelli V, et al. Reproductive performance before and after myomectomy: a retrospective analysis. Fertil Steril. 2004;82(1):154-9.
20. Goldenberg M, Sivan E, Sharabi Z, et al. Outcome of hysteroscopic resection of submucous myomas for infertility. Fertil Steril. 1995;64(4):714-6.
21. Yanaihara A, Yorimitsu T, Motoyama H, et al. Location of the endometrial polyp and its pregnancy rate of infertility patients. Fertil Steril. 2007;88 Suppl 1:S191-2.
22. Stamatellos I, Apostolides A, Stamatopoulos P, et al. Pregnancy rates after hysteroscopic polypectomy depending on the size or number of the polyps. Arch Gynecol Obstet. 2008;277(5):395-9.
23. Murad K. Spontaneous Pregnancy Following Ulipristal Acetate Treatment in a Woman with a Symptomatic Uterine Fibroid. J Obstet Gynaecol Can. 2016;38(1):75-9.
24. Schenker JG, Margalioth EJ. Intrauterine adhesions: an updated appraisal. Fertil Steril. 1982;37 (5):593-610.
25. Kodaman PH, Arici A. Intra-uterine adhesions and fertility outcome: how to optimize success? Curr Opin Obstet Gynecol. 2007;19(3):207-14.
26. Lotgering FK. Clinical aspects of cervical insufficiency. BMC Pregnancy Childbirth. 2007;7(Suppl 1):S17.
27. Mastrolia SA, Baumfeld Y, Hershkovitz R, et al. Bicornuate uterus is an independent risk factor for cervical os insufficiency: A retrospective population based cohort study. J Matern Fetal Neonatal Med. 2017;30(22):2705-10.
28. Miller ES, Gerber SE. Association between sonographic cervical appearance and preterm delivery after a history-indicated cerclage. J Ultrasound Med. 2014;33(12):2181-6.
29. Bohîlțea RE, Munteanu O, Turcan N, et al. A debate about ultrasound and anatomic aspects of the cervix in spontaneous preterm birth. J Med Life. 2016;9(4):342-7.
30. Crosby DA, Miletin J, Semberova J, et al. Is routine transvaginal cervical length measurement cost-effective in a population where the

risk of spontaneous preterm birth is low? Acta Obstet Gynecol Scand. 2016;95(12):1391-5.
31. Berghella V, Baxter JK, Hendrix NW. Cervical assessment by ultrasound for preventing preterm delivery. Cochrane Database Syst Rev. 2009;(3):CD007235.
32. Fox NS, Chervenak FA. Cervical cerclage: a review of the evidence. Obstet Gynecol Surv. 2008; 63(1):58-65.
33. Drakeley AJ, Roberts D, Alfirevic Z. Cervical stitch (cerclage) for preventing pregnancy loss in women. Cochrane Database Syst Rev. 2003;(1):CD003253.
34. Final report of the Medical Research Council/Royal College of Obstetricians and Gynaecologists multicentre randomised trial of cervical cerclage. MRC/RCOG Working Party on Cervical Cerclage. Br J Obstet Gynaecol. 1993;100(6):516-23.

Chapter 4

Immunology of Recurrent Pregnancy Miscarriage

INTRODUCTION

It is now well established that recurrent spontaneous miscarriages of immunological origin are one more manifestation of obstetric vasculopathies. In simplest terms, obstetric vasculopathy means disease of vessels resulting from an obstetric event. Though this is the first step to the understanding of obstetric vasculopathies, it is the simplest and most preliminary step. Immediately from here the complexity of this science begins. It is indeed this complexity that makes it very beautiful but challenging, intriguing, and therefore inviting for its keen students to decode its mysteries.

Obstetric vasculopathy is not the vasculopathy that occurs in the maternal vascular system. It is the vasculopathy that occurs at the fetomaternal interface. Inherited probably by the genetic propensity at the fetomaternal system, there occurs a series of changed at this interface which invites seemingly totally diverse and apparently unrelated conditions.

In early understandings, it was perceived that one condition leads to the other. But as advances in understanding increased it became obvious that this is not a cause-effect relationship but are fruits of the same pathology. In the initial years, only a few conditions were attributed to obstetric vasculopathy, viz.:
- Recurrent spontaneous miscarriages
- Intrauterine growth retardations (IUGRs)
- Preeclampsia (PE) and PE remote from term
- Accidental hemorrhage
- Chorea gravidarum.

However, with scientific research going in details of these conditions, more specifics and complexities added up. Currently, obstetric vasculopathies include:
- Recurrent spontaneous missed abortions of late 1st trimesters and 2nd trimesters.
- Accidental hemorrhage with association of IUGR or PE remote from term.
- Fetal demise of nonanomalous pregnancies with an association of any one of the earlier conditions.

With the etiopathology becoming clearer, it has become clear that the differentiation of PE remote from term from PE was unnecessary. It was, therefore, subsequently dropped.

HYPERHOMOCYSTEINEMIA AND RECURRENT MISCARRIAGE

Hyperhomocysteinemia is a relatively newer addition in the field of understanding of recurrent spontaneous miscarriage. Homocysteine (Hcy) is a sulfur-containing amino acid produced when methionine is demethylated. The majority of Hcy undergoes transsulfuration to cysteine by cystathionine beta-synthase (CBS), of which vitamin B6 (pyridoxine) is an essential cofactor. The remainder of Hcy is remethylated by methionine synthase (MS), of which vitamin B12 (cobalamin) is an essential cofactor along with methylenetetrahydrofolate (MTHF). MTHF is generated by the enzyme MTHF reductase (MTHFR). High levels of Hcy can result from a variety of acquired factors (deficiency of vitamins B6, B12 and folic acid, high meat diet, smoking, and others) or genetic (abnormalities of methionine-Hcy metabolism). Hyperhomocysteinemia is associated with premature atherosclerosis and venous thromboembolism, so called "cholesterol of XXI age". Results of many studies suggest that hyperhomocysteinemia, homozygous state for MTHFR gene mutation, and folate deficiency are probably risk factors for recurrent fetal loss, intrauterine fetal death, thromboembolic disease in pregnancy, neural tube defects and congenital cardiac malformation at infants, and other placental conditions (PE, placental abruption, and IUGR). The plasma Hcy values can be modulated by vitamins, vitamin B6, and folic acid in particular.[1]

SYSTEMIC LUPUS ERYTHEMATOSUS

Systemic lupus erythematosus (SLE) associated pregnancies are an individual class. They have a magnified manifestation of vasculopathy thereby enabling a closer look at this miraculous but mysterious phenomenon. It needs to be clarified here that all obstetric vasculopathies are not SLE but SLE does produce obstetric vasculopathy. Also, immunology and its disturbances have a significant role to play in obstetric vasculopathy. These aspects will be handled in details in the following pages of this chapter.

LEADS FOR OBSTETRIC VASCULOPATHIES THROUGH RECURRENT SPONTANEOUS ABORTION

There are explainable and unexplainable causes of recurrent spontaneous abortion (RSA). The classic example of explainable causes includes the anatomical defects of the genital tract, both congenital and acquired. However, the most intriguing and therefore the most challenging among all causes remain immunological causes. They are very complicated to understand and a test to treat. Nevertheless, they prove very vital leads to the understanding of obstetric vasculopathy.

FETUS AS AN ALLOGRAFT

It is well understood that the fetus is immunologically a very dynamic structure. It bears an expression of maternal as well as paternal antigens on itself. Any foreign protein that enters a human body generates a series of immunological reactions in the host. These are the responses that ultimately destroy the entrant to protect the host. On these very lines, the fetus is also a graft, albeit an allograft that is transplanted into the mother's body. It has in itself an expression of maternal and paternal alloantigens. The fetus, therefore, behaves as a transplanted graft. It has been a big challenge for all transplant scientists to understand how does the fetus quiescence the host reaction and generates a peaceful acceptance. This phenomenon is the key to any graft acceptance.

There is no reason why the fetus also should not be treated as a graft. Attempts are bound to be made by the maternal immune system to reject it. The paternal alloantigens are foreign to the maternal immune system. They generate the graft-host reaction. The maternal antigens are not alien to the mother. They are her own. Therefore, the mother accepts those antigens. But the paternal antigens have no business to expect such a warm welcome and tolerance by the mother's system.

Now that it has been understood that the fetus is an allograft which too has an expression of antigens, the question that arises is why does the fetus escape from the rejection phenomenon? Not only does the fetus not get rejected but it is also made to thrive and is nourished. On one side are the protective mechanisms in the mother that readily reject any foreign graft and on the other are the maternal system that tolerates, accepts, nourishes, and ensures that the fetal allograft thrives. What provides this privileged status to the fetus? How does this miracle occur? The antigens that have been found to have a significant bearing on this entire phenomenon are the antigens of the major histocompatibility complex (MHC). These antibodies have been documented to bind the cells of the fetus and the trophoblast.

What Protects the Fetus?

Due to ethical constraints, most of the understanding of human pregnancy and the immunological response comes from studies in mice. Mice too have a hemochorial pregnancy and are therefore providing valuable insight into the understanding of human pregnancy tolerance.

Small Size

The small size of the embryo does help in protecting it. The effector cells from the maternal system that may have strayed into the fallopian tube or the peritoneal pelvic fluid fail to detect this small embryo. Also, due to this small size, there is no interaction between the maternal lymphatic systems and the embryo. This small size also prevents the detection of the embryo while it transits from the fallopian tube to the uterus. Hill (1987) demonstrated that if for whatever reason, the macrophage effector cell system does get activated; it effectively releases destructive cytokines like tumor necrosis factor-alpha (TNF-α) and granulocyte-macrophage colony-stimulating factor (GM-CSF), interleukin-1, interleukin-6, and others.[2] It can lead to implantation failure following embryo damage. The fact that these inflammatory substances do play a critical role in protection–destruction interplay of the fetal allograft has been demonstrated in another study in which it was found that for the first time that allograft inflammatory factor-1 (AIF-1) was expressed in uterus. The expression level was associated with the population size of macrophage and varied during the estrous cycle and the pregnancy period. The augmented expression of AIF-1 with concomitant expressions of TNF-α and nitric oxide synthase 2 (NOS2) messenger ribonucleic acid (mRNA) in poly (I:C) injected mice suggests a correlation between AIF-1 production and fetal resorption.[3]

Zona Pellucida

The shield provided by the zona pellucida plays a treasured role in the failure of the maternal protective system while the embryo is in its phase of transit migration. It is not precisely understood as to whether the zona provides a physical barrier to the detection by the maternal protective systems only or also makes the embryo hypoantigenic. The role of zona in protecting the conceptus is confined to the transit. It is proved by it getting shed off just before implantation. It is not required once the embryo reaches the uterus. One study has shown that the zona pellucida thickness has a significant influence on in vivo fertilization and implantation processes, but not on birth.[4]

Paralysis of Maternal Protector Systems and Pregnancy

In the days when hysterosalpingography and Rubin's tubal insufflation tests were still attractive for tubal patency testing, clinicians know that there used to be successful pregnancies just after performing these tests. This phenomenon was more consistently observed after hysterosalpingography and is attributed to the transient paralysis or ablation of maternal macrophage effectors systems. This is the explanation to how the fetal embryo gets protected in transit. However, the bigger challenge lies in protecting, implanting, and bringing about a thriving growth of the conceptus.

Hypoimmunogenic Embryo

The mechanisms of protection of embryo from getting destroyed by the maternal protective systems also include its hypoimmunogenicity. The embryo is always flat in creating an immune reaction. As it has been stated in previous pages, there are different types of antigens expressing on its surface. These include products of the MHC or major histocompatibility complex (H) such as human leukocyte antigen (HLA) and non-MHC or minor histocompatibility (h) gene complexes. It is interesting to note that expression of (H) is shut off before implantation. This process is an important change in the embryo to render it hypoantigenic.[5]

It seems the hormone leptin, which is primarily produced by adipose tissue, is a critical permissive factor for multiple reproductive events (in the mouse), including implantation. Throughout development, leptin patterning suggests that it is a component of the subcortical maternal complex with as yet unknown significance in preimplantation development.[6]

Fetus as a Unique Allograft

A question arises in the investigators mind as to why does the fetus not get rejected. It is extremely complicated but fascinating phenomenon. The conceptus has two mechanisms of immunologically active strata. One is the fetus itself, and the other is the trophoblast. The fetal tissue is immunologically susceptible to recognition and rejection by the mother. This rejection would occur if there is a direct interaction between the fetal surface and the maternal lymphomyeloid cells. In animal experiments, it has been found that if the fetal tissue is directly injected into the thigh of mice, there is an immediate rejection of this tissue.[7] Direct contact between the maternal lymphocytes and fetal cells can also occur if there is an intrauterine transfusion accidentally or spontaneously. This contact leads to fetal rejection.

Entry of maternal cells in fetal circulation and entry of fetal cells into the maternal system is rare. But the maternal system has a significant advantage. It has a very competent effector system, and the intruding fetal cells are quickly and efficiently eliminated from the maternal protective system. If in any instance there is a failure of any of these systems graft-versus-host (GVH) diseases get manifested.

On the flip side, the phenomenon of fetal microchimerism has been found to have interesting bearings. Fetal cells can persist in a wide range of woman's tissues following a pregnancy or a miscarriage, and she becomes a chimera. Fetal cells have been found in the maternal circulation, and they were shown to persist for the entire life in humans, thus demonstrating long-term engraftment and survival capabilities. Microchimerism is a subject of much interest for a number of reasons. Studies of fetal microchimerism during pregnancy may offer explanations for complications of pregnancy, such as PE, as well as insights into the pathogenesis of autoimmune diseases which usually ameliorate during pregnancy. The impact of the persistence of allogeneic cells of fetal origin and the maternal immunological response to them on the mother's health is still not clear. On the beneficial side, it has been proposed that genetically dissimilar fetal microchimerism protects against some cancers, that fetal microchimerism can afford the mother new mechanisms of protection to some diseases, that fetal microchimerism can enlarge the immunological range of the mother improving her defense against the aggressor. Fetal cells are often present at sites of maternal injury and may have an active role in the repair of maternal tissues.[8]

Now let us see a very intriguing phenomenon. The estimated instance of the passage of maternal lymphocytes is believed to be rare but at 1 in 50 to 1 in 100 embryos. We have seen that if at any instance such an exchange if at all it occurs, the fetus gets rejected. Thus, the estimated spontaneous resorption rate (in mice) and miscarriage rate in humans should be around 1–2% (1 in 50 to 1 in 100). But in actual clinical practice, this rate is much higher. Thus, there is some more to explain than mere lymphocytes of the mother playing havoc.

This is where the second strata of immunological activity beyond the conceptus steps and this layer is the stratum of trophoblasts. It is well established since the mid-1980s that the trophoblasts are very specialized forms of tissues as regards genetic expression is concerned. There are two groups: One that is found primarily at the fetomaternal interface between the fetoplacental capillaries and maternal blood (fetal interface), the second is at the maternal interface in contact with the decidua.

Fetal trophoblasts are substantially dependent on paternal genetic material for their survival and development. However, if there is only paternal genetic material pathological pregnancies like gestational trophoblastic diseases develop. It means that the maternal genetic expression on the trophoblast helps in creating a balance. It is well known that there is an uncontrolled growth of trophoblastic tissue in hydatidiform mole. This uncontrolled growth is checked by the expression of maternal genetic material on trophoblast which brings about a healthy fetal growth and development.

It is fascinating to note that in the absence of maternal genetic expression the trophoblasts have a field day. This paradox is worth understanding. The maternal immune system is derived from the mother and therefore should not give any resistance to growth or survival of its own material. However, the paternal contribution is alien to the maternal effector system. The latter is supposed to react and protect the maternal system by eliminating any foreign genetic material. Nevertheless, at the fetomaternal interface, a complete reversal of this phenomenon occurs. Instead of removing the tissue with paternal genetic expression (alien to the mother), it brings about a growth of these trophoblasts.

A complete foreign or alien genetic material seems to promote trophoblastic growth. Only paternal genetic expression, however, brings about uncontrolled growth as is seen in hydatidiform mole. It appears that such an uncontrolled growth is prevented by the maternal genetic material. Thus, at the level of the trophoblast, an entirely paradoxical situation develops. Foreign genetic material promotes growth and genetic material from the host check this growth or may even hamper this growth. It seems that the trophoblast has a privileged status. This privileged status is given to the syncytiotrophoblasts.

An important characteristic of most trophoblasts is their capacity to resist rejection by the host antigen specific effectors mechanism. This privileged status of the trophoblast is the key to the survival and growth of a partly foreign genetic material on the conceptus in an alien environment (the maternal environment).

The early invasion of the trophoblast into the maternal spiral arterioles and their resistance to maternal elimination systems are the keys to healthy pregnancy outcome. As a corollary to this, any impendence or failure to this invasion can lead to complete rejection of fetal tissue. This phenomenon is seen in miscarriages. In subjects in whom the trophoblasts partially resist maternal rejection, manifestations of other obstetric vasculopathies result. Thus, pregnancy-induced hypertension (PIH) and IUGR are a result of partial rejection by the host.

Hence, it gets well established that paternal genetic expression is the key to the survival of fetal tissue. It is the paternal genetic material which is the growth driver in the trophoblast and subsequently in the fetus. The trophoblasts are extremely resistant to maternal rejection due to a paternal genetic expression which is a privileged status. This resistance is intrinsic.

The entire spectrum of healthy fetal growth and development along with resistance to rejection gets explained. At one end of the spectrum is a total failure of trophoblast to resist the maternal rejection systems. It results in a miscarriage. At the middle of the spectrum is an array of obstetric vasculopathies where there is a partial rejection or partial activation of maternal effectors systems not killing the conceptus but producing diseased states. On the other extreme of the spectrum is a hydatidiform mole. In this, there is only paternal genetic expression and no maternal expression. It gives a field day to the trophoblasts leading to their uncontrolled growth. Therefore, there is a strong genetic platform for the immunological basis for obstetric vasculopathies. These will be revisited in the pages to follow.

Suppressor Mechanisms in Protection

In this section, we shall see one more unique and unusual phenomenon that takes place at the level of the decidua which plays a significant role in the successful nidation and then a proper growth of the fetus. At this stage, it will be worthwhile noting that all these protective mechanisms act partly in tandem with each other and partially independent to achieve the ultimate goal of a successful pregnancy outcome. Scrupulous understanding of these mechanisms will play a pivotal role in our understanding of the processes involved in causation, and management of obstetric vasculopathies.

Just before implantation, workers like Brierley and Clark and Daya et al. have shown that unique populations of cells develop in the uterine lining. These are the suppressor cells. They are unique in ways more than one. They are developed under the hormonal influence and not under the influence of antigens. They are locally generated, confining themselves to the uterine lining, and not all across the mother's body. They are relatively large cells resembling the structure and function of T cells.[9,10] To understand the role of suppressor T cells, one has to know the concepts of DTH or delayed type of hypersensitivity reaction. If DTH is generated before the time, it can prove lethal to the process of successful implantation. However, the same process of DTH is necessary later to maintain a proper growth of the conceptus postimplantation.

Now let us see why these suppressor T cells get generated in the uterine lining. Firstly, they have a capacity to keep the maternal macrophages at bay. Secondly, they delay the generation of DTH preventing its occurrence in first 4 days. If DTH occurs as early as the first day of implantation, it will sense an allergen-like antigen in the implanting conceptus. This premature sensing will bring about changes to cause its rejection. It also includes activating macrophages. Whether the suppressor T cells can keep the macrophages at bay individually or through the delay in generation of DTH is not known.

By the fifth postimplantation day, these large T-cell suppressors get replaced by smaller suppressor cell population. This replacement is necessary as the new population of cells has a different role to play besides protecting the conceptus. They also have a function to generate potent immunological molecule RGF-B which promotes new blood vessel formation and growth. These are early steps being taken to generate a healthy growth of the conceptus.

Before we go further into the depth of understanding the role of these new suppressor cells, we need to revise some basic facts. The conceptus is half alien to the mother. Therefore, the tendency of the maternal protecting systems to reject and eliminate it is understandable. Through a series of complicated but amazing mechanisms, the conceptus protects itself from getting eliminated. At the same time, the maternal protective systems help the conceptus to successfully implant and then nidate and grow.

To understand this complex phenomenon a little more easily, one can draw a parallel in something that is occurring in the world, so naturally. Every large and thriving country has a problem of illegal migrants. India too has such a problem. Simplistically put, the conceptus is such an illegal migrant. Illegal immigrants devise different mechanisms by which sneak in through the Indian borders. To avoid detection, it may sneak in at night or through porous areas on the Indian borders. Once within the territory of India, politicians who may have been bribed or may have same political ulterior motives generate mechanisms by which this migrant gets some foothold either at some shanty dwelling or as a guest of some host without getting detected. Soon the politician becomes his protector and generates illegal housing, ration benefits and subsequently even gets him a voting right. The migrant under the patronage of his protector soon starts getting accepted in his new country. He starts growing in acceptance, starts his own business, or gets some other employment. As time passes, he grows so much in stature that even becomes an accepted leader thereby influencing the entire host mechanism in its favor.

The fetus also behaves similarly. As pregnancy advances, it grows in size and maturity and changes the whole maternal physiology in such a way that it may even endanger the mother's life to ensure its survival. This newly generated smaller suppressor cell crop can suppress destruction of the embryo by releasing a potent immune suppressive molecule like transforming growth factor-beta (TGF-β).

This molecule seems to be inhibitive to natural killer (NK) cells and suppresses the plethora of destructive cytokines like interleukin-3 (IL-3). Thus, this TGF-β appears to have a potent capacity to block nearly all maternal effectors systems.[11,12]

It seems that TGF-β and TNF-α has a point to point antagonizing mechanism as regards to their effects on immune mechanisms.[13] While one protects and prepares for the growth and development of the conceptus, the other is a potent protector of the mother. TNF-α is all out to destroy any immunologically alien molecule, in this case, the conceptus. It gets neutralized by TGF-β.

From a bird's eye view, it seems the general opinion is that the fundamental protective mechanism must be located locally on the contact plate, between the maternal and fetal tissues. Immunologic investigations proved the presence of specific systems which block the function of antipaternal maternal antibodies, as well as the formation of cytotoxic maternal T-cells to paternal antigens. The system preventing rejection of graft during pregnancy is operating at the level of maternal and fetal tissues. The protective mechanisms are coded by genes of MHC region, locus HLA-G.

Protective Mechanisms in the Placenta

The placenta protects itself against antibody-mediated damage. High levels of complement regulatory proteins (CD46, CD55, and CD59) are produced in response to the synthesis of complement fixing maternal antibodies to paternal antigens. Regulation of the placental HLA expression as a defensive reaction of the fetoplacental unit to the influence of protective cytotoxic T lymphocytes (CTLs) is the most important protective mechanisms of the placenta.

Protective Mechanisms Shared by the Placenta and Uterus

Protective mechanisms common both for placenta and uterus are as follows: Expressions of Fas ligand, prevention of infiltration of activated immune cells, regulation of immunosuppression which prevents the proliferation of immune cells, and high natural immunity (Na cells and macrophages) of the decidua.[14]

PARTNER SPECIFICITY IN MISCARRIAGES

In the early 90s, there was a trend to classify women who abort as primary aborters and secondary aborters. Primary aborters were those mothers who aborted all her pregnancies and never had a successful outcome. On the other hand, secondary aborters were those who at some time or the other have had at least one successful outcome. By successful outcome, it was meant as a live birth. Interestingly primary miscarriages seemed to be partner specific and secondary aborters, aborted irrespective of the partner. Though this classification did not become clinically popular, it raised some interesting questions.

It is possible that partner specific miscarriages could have a genetic basis, but nonpartner specific miscarriages have an explanation beyond the faulty genetic material. Currently, it is accepted that majority of miscarriages result from immunological problems. This issue can be simply worded as failure to prevent rejection. It is fascinating to note that 25% of mothers threaten a miscarriage, but only 10% actually abort. It means that while the maternal system is all out to reject it (threatened abortion), the fetal system protects itself from the rejection onslaught and successful outcome results. If fetal heart activity can be detected in the 1st trimester more than 90%, conceptuses gestate successfully. Thus, the onus of initial survival of the fetus against the maternal onslaught is not on the shoulders of the mother but in the fetus itself.

Also, the clinical phenomenon of threatened miscarriage is merely a clinical expression of the ongoing conflict between the fetal system to survive and the maternal system to destroy. As it has been hinted in some of the preceding pages cytokines have a vital role to play in this process. It is well known that there are a set of protective cytokines and destructive cytokines. This activity occurs throughout the maternal vascular channels. As a result of this, there is an injury and rupture of the vascular system resulting in threatened miscarriage clinically.

However, it is not necessary that the destructive cytokines should win or lose. The war may go on any side. If the destructive cytokines win, the mother aborts. If protective cytokines win, it results in a favorable outcome. But this entire process mediates through the vascular bed irrespective of the result. As a result, threatened miscarriage is far more prevalent than an actual miscarriage. This complex interplay of cytokines is tackled separately in sections to follow.

While the trophoblasts have an intrinsic capacity to resist maternal immunologic destruction, it should be noted that a certain immune response associated (IA) antigens have an important role to play in this. This IA antigens associate with a variety of foreign molecules and allow their recognition by T-helper/delayed-type hypersensitivity (DTH) cells. Animals deficient in IA antigens cannot mount an immune response to defined epitopes.

The gene coding of IA genes has been called as immune response genes. A difference in IA expression causes maximum proliferation of responding T cells.[15] Interestingly these IA antigens are absent on the trophoblast. It could be one of the mechanisms by which the trophoblasts resist maternal destruction responses.

Of late, the roles of HLA and MCHs in human pregnancy have been found to be limited. The other responses though similar are equally interesting and intriguing. It has been suggested by proponents of HLA sharing hypothesis that recurrent miscarriage represents a heterogeneous group of subjects and this sharing is relevant only to a subgroup.[15] In that case, the two primary subgroups proposed are:

1. *Primary aborters:* They abort with one partner and have a significant HLA sharing. They have no live births.
2. *Secondary aborters:* They have one or more live births, no HLA sharing, may abort with several partners, and may possess antibodies to paternal cells.[12]

All these mechanisms of immune recognition, tolerance, and rejection play a significant role in recurrent miscarriages due to immune causes.

Primary Aborters and Nonimmunological Basis

By and large discussion on primary and secondary aborters hover around immunological basis for the same. However, there are some who believe that primary aborters may have a predisposition for maternal meiosis errors resulting in digyny. Digyny (also digynia) refers to the process of a diploid ovum becoming fertilized by a monoploid sperm. The result of digyny is a triploid zygote. A case report supporting the concept that some women have a predisposition for maternal meiosis errors resulting in digyny have also been published.[16] Similarly, anatomical corrections have also ended in successful pregnancy outcome in primary aborters. There is a report where septoplasty allowed successful delivery in a primary aborter with six previous 1st trimester miscarriages.[17] It would, therefore, be wise if these rarer occurrences are kept in mind while one evaluates a subject of recurrent miscarriages before attributing all of them to obstetric vasculopathy.

AUTOIMMUNITY IN RECURRENT PREGNANCY LOSS

A smaller but significant group associated with obstetric vasculopathy is that of autoantibodies. Among a variety of autoantibodies that have been found to have an association with obstetric vasculopathies, antiphospholipid (APL) antibodies have been found to have the most consistent and reproducible association.

Antiphospholipid Antibodies

Antiphospholipid syndrome (APS) is a systemic autoimmune disease characterized by vascular thrombosis (arterial or venous) and pregnancy complications associated with the occurrence of autoantibodies. These autoantibodies specifically include lupus anticoagulant, anticardiolipin antibodies, and/or anti-β2 glycoprotein-I (anti-β2GPI) antibodies. According to the 2006 Sydney criteria, it is recommended that these antibodies should be confirmed at least twice over a 12-weeks period.[18,19] APL antibodies are a diverse group of antibodies that were first described by Wassermann as early as in 1906. But it was only in 1952 that Country and Hartman described them in patients with SLE. Soon it became apparent that APL antibodies can exist without any connective tissue disorders. These are a diverse family of autoantibodies which share a common reactivity with negatively charged phospholipids.

Many members have been described to constitute the group of APL antibodies. Of these only three have been found to have a clinical bearing.

These are:
1. Biological false seropositive for syphilis (BFSPS)
2. Anticardiolipin antibodies (ACAs)
3. Lupus anticoagulant (LAC).

A word regarding BFSPS: The reactivity of serum of many patients of recurrent miscarriages to phospholipids falsely testing positive for syphilis was intriguing. Many subjects tested positive for syphilis did not have any other stigma of syphilis. It brought two facts to light: (1) These subjects never had syphilis and (2) They had a consistent adverse obstetric outcome.

Lupus anticoagulant or LAC antibodies are autoantibodies which prolong phospholipids dependent coagulation assays by reacting with negatively charged phospholipids. Interestingly while LAC has been associated with SLE, they are more often than not found in subjects without SLE. Most of these patients have only manifestations of obstetric vasculopathies without any association with SLE. Anticardiolipin antibodies or ACA as they are popularly known are so named because these groups of antibodies were initially extracted from bovine heart tissue.

Role of a Cofactor

In early 1990s, workers like Matsuura had evinced interest in the role and need of a cofactor in the activity of ACAs in obstetric vasculopathies.[20] It seems that the anticardiolipin (ACL) antibodies when released from a result of an infection like syphilis behave differently than those released out of an autoimmune process. Whereas the ACL antibodies of autoimmune origin need a cofactor for its activity, ACL antibodies released from other sources do not need a cofactor. This cofactor has been identified as β2-glycoprotein 1 (β2GP1).[21]

It was postulated that the cofactor β2GP1 may:
- Inhibit intrinsic phase of coagulation
- May inhibit platelet activation and
- It is an APL binding protein.

These three processes are critical in the causation of obstetric vasculopathies.

Prevalence of Antiphospholipid

Calculating prevalence is an interesting aspect of the autoantibodies. In general population also APL antibodies have been demonstrated. But in all of these, obstetric vasculopathy did not occur. Around this time association between APA and PE remote from term was investigated by us and we found that 53.3% of subjects tested positive. Of these, low positive were 17.9%, moderate positive were 50.0%, and strong positive were 32.1%.[22] It is understood that low levels of APL antibodies are important to cause obstetric vasculopathies. Therefore, when the cutout values are higher, a significant association with obstetric vasculopathies can occur. It means that a mere presence of APL antibodies at low levels do not have a much clinical bearing. Therefore, mere presence of APL antibodies is not an indication for starting any treatment. Case-controlled studies have also demonstrated that APL antibodies have a direct influence in causation of obstetric vasculopathies.[23]

However, the study by Infante-Rivard needs a special mention. This study which did not show such an association suffered from a handicap. These workers had included single miscarriage also in their study. It proved two points: (1) Single miscarriages are not associated with APL and (2) The study got diluted by this inclusion of single miscarriages and therefore, became less reliable.[24]

Pathogenesis

The primary problematic nucleus for obstetric vasculopathy is at the fetomaternal interface. As in its alloimmune counterpart, in autoimmune causes of obstetric vasculopathies also the underlying mischief occurs at the level of the placenta. In a normal physiological change of pregnancy, the trophoblasts invade the maternal spiral arterioles. They destroy the arteriolar intima and replace the endothelial cell lining. Thus, there is a conversion of the fetomaternal interface to a low resistance pool of blood which is critical to the development of a healthy pregnancy.

Under the effect of APL antibodies, these changes do not occur. Instead of a destruction of the muscular and elastic tissue by the invading trophoblasts, the vessels get loaded by the immune complex deposits after decidual necrosis. The vascular bed, in that case, fails to form the low resistance pool of blood. In actuality, it becomes a high resistance point impoverished of efficient blood supply. The conceptus fails to get nourished resulting into a series of adverse obstetric outcomes. All these are grouped as obstetric vasculopathies. In early phases of pregnancy there is a miscarriage, in late pregnancy there is IUGR. Besides these, the obstetric vasculopathies also include PIH, accidental hemorrhage, and fetal death.

Platelets

Having understood the effect of APL antibodies on the vessel walls at fetomaternal interface, it would now be worthwhile examining the role of APL antibodies on other cells and tissues. These effects may not be principally acting to cause obstetric vasculopathies but contribute in some way to same. Among these, the effect on platelets has been studied in details. It has been found that APL antibodies do not affect inactivated platelets. But they bind with activated platelets. Phospholipids are found to have been distributed at the platelet cell membranes when activated. They cause a local dysfunction of hemostatic mechanism which is critical for proper placentation and maintenance of healthy pregnancy.

Although underestimated, platelets may be involved in APS and its thrombotic manifestations, mainly arterial, in several ways. Thrombocytopenia is the most important manifestation of APS, possibly caused by direct binding of anti-β2GPI antibodies or anti-β2-GPI-β2-GPI complexes. On the other hand, platelets may have a fundamental role in APS-related thrombosis. This role may be due to the presence of multiple receptors that can interact with anti-β2GPI antibodies especially apolipoprotein E-receptor-2' (apoER2') and glycoprotein Ibα (GPIbα). It leads to a consequent release of different procoagulant mediators such as thromboxane B2, platelet factor 4 (PF4), and platelet factor 4 variant (CXCL4L1).[25]

Disruption of Thromboxane Prostacyclin Mechanism

For normal caliber and proper perfusion of the maternal vascular system, a balance between prostacyclin thromboxane activities is critical. During normal pregnancy, there is a bias of the balance to tilt towards vasodilatory system prostacyclin. Though some disruption seems to be occurring in the prostacyclin thromboxane balance system in the presence of APL antibodies to what extent it produces the consequences of obstetric vasculopathies is a matter of conjecture.

Protein C Activation

One more mechanism by which APL antibodies may be acting is by activation of protein C. A protein present on the vascular endothelium called thrombomodulin helps to achieve this. This protein has to be bound to phospholipids for activation of protein C. In some subjects APL antibodies inhibit this mechanism. Also for its activity protein C needs a cofactor known as protein S. It has been found that once bound to platelet membranes, the protein C-protein S complex inhibits coagulation factors Va and Xa. This activity is inhibited by APL antibodies. However, this effect has not been consistently found suggesting that it is prevalent only in some subjects with obstetric vasculopathy. Thus, the primary mechanism of APL activity is the action on the vascular bed directly as it has been stated in preceding pages. Through this, the APL antibodies prevent the destruction of vascular intima and elastin so critical for vascular modulation. At the same time, other mechanisms just act as adjuvants to this primary mechanism.

Is there a Crossover between Different Antiphospholipid (APL) Antibodies?

It is interesting to note how advances in science refine the understanding of various disease processes. In early and mid-1990s it was thought that there is a considerable crossover between three main types of APL antibodies of clinical importance, viz.:
1. Anticardiolipin antibodies
2. Lupus anticoagulant and
3. Biological false seropositive for syphilis antibodies.

However, in early 2000 it was found that such crossover does not exist. Therefore, if a clinician or a scientist wants to investigate a subject of obstetric vasculopathy for an autoimmune association, it will be necessary for them to assess both—ACL antibodies as well as LAC in any particular subject. Initially, it was thought that only ACL antibody assessment would suffice. But in 2005 it was found that both need to be assessed. In the absence of any clinical, it leads to suspect syphilis assessment of BFPS that is not of use in subjects with obstetric vasculopathies.

Interestingly there is one study that examined midluteal phase uterine artery blood flow through Doppler assessment in nonpregnant women having a history of recurrent spontaneous miscarriages. It was found that uterine arteries pulsatility index (PI) values in RSA patients were significantly higher concerning those found in the control group. When patients were grouped according to the different RSA causes, the highest PI values were observed among patients with uterine abnormalities, APL antibodies syndrome, and unexplained RSA in that order. The authors suggested that increased resistance to uterine blood flow may be an important contributing factor to some causes of RSA and may represent an independent indication of the risk of pregnancy loss.[26]

Other Contributory Mechanisms

Antiphospholipid antibodies seem to generate some other changes in vivo to produce a hostile environment for the fetus. One of them is a failure to block complement activation. Complements like C3 and

C4 have been found to play a significant role in protecting the host by destroying the foreign graft. In a successful pregnancy implantation and growth, maternal protecting mechanisms need to be blunted. APL antibodies generate such environments that the complement C3 and C4 activation are blunted. Once C3 and C4 get activated the intrauterine environment becomes hostile to the trophoblasts, and a destruction of efficient trophoblastic invasion occurs. This process leads to a destruction of the fetal graft and clinically manifests as missed abortion.

Defective Generation of Syncytiotrophoblasts

Syncytiotrophoblasts are the key trophoblasts that protect the fetus graft from getting rejected. These syncytiotrophoblasts are privileged cell linings that have a series of defense mechanisms that prevent the fetus from getting rejected. One of the ways by which the alloimmune or autoimmune mechanism of obstetric vasculopathies occurs is a failure to generate competent syncytiotrophoblasts. As it is well known, cytotrophoblasts fuse with one another to create this specialized syncytiotrophoblasts lining.

Trophoblast molecules like integrin and cadherin have an important role to play in this generation of defective syncytiotrophoblasts. There are two types of integrins: (1) One that inhibits trophoblastic invasion like In-1 and (2) Others that promote trophoblastic invasion like In-5.

Cadherins (named for *calcium-dependent adhesion*) are a class of type 1 transmembrane proteins. They play an important role in cell adhesion, ensuring that cells within tissues are bound together. They are dependent on calcium (Ca^{++}) ions to function, hence their name. The cadherin superfamily includes cadherins, protocadherins, desmogleins and desmocollins, and more. In structure, they share cadherin repeats, which are the extracellular Ca^{++}-binding domains. There are multiple classes of cadherin molecule, each designated with a prefix (in general, noting the type of tissue with which it is associated). It has been observed that cells containing a particular cadherin subtype tend to cluster together to the exclusion of other types, both in cell culture and during development.[27]

Cadherin VE and cadherin E are two subtypes of the large family of cadherins that cause an efficient fusion of cytotrophoblasts leading to a genesis of competent and efficient syncytiotrophoblasts. These two cadherin subtypes are believed to have a significant role in aggregation, differentiation, and subsequent fusion of cytotrophoblasts. These three phenomena subsequently result in the generation of competent syncytiotrophoblasts.[27]

It seems that APL antibodies immunoglobulin G (IgG) cause a downregulation of VE cadherin and upregulation of E cadherin. This downregulation induces refractoriness to productive cadherin activity which ultimately leads to failure of one or all three mechanisms needed for the genesis of competent syncytiotrophoblasts.

Incompetent Gonadotropin-releasing Hormone Activity

Besides the complex link between the immunology and genetics in successful pregnancy outcome, endocrinal components are also having a key role to play in this process of trophoblastic activity. Gonadotropin-releasing hormone (GnRH) is the step where immunological failures may be occurring. APL antibodies blunt the GnRH activity thereby disturbing the healthy hormonal milieu that is required for promoting a healthy pregnancy foundation.

Privileged Status of Syncytiotrophoblasts

One of the most intriguing phenomena that occur in the human body in particular and in the entire living kingdom, in general, is the phenomenon of reproduction. Furthermore, in this process of reproduction, the array of changes that take place to allow the fetus allograft to be tolerated, kept alive, and nourished is still more intriguing and even sometimes a scary phenomenon. Not a single step in this is simple. Offering simplistic explanations to these would amount to bordering inexactitudes.

In the society, mothers are supposed to be most loving and most protective about her children. But in the process of reproduction, she consistently and continuously tries to destroy the fetus allograft. This behavior of her protective systems should not come as a surprise because the fetus has immunologically two components: (1) The component from the mother and (2) The component from the father. The fetal immunological component that has been received from the mother is her own. This component is innate to her. As a result, she has no problems in tolerating this component. However, the paternal component is immunologically alien to her. It is a foreign protein. Universally, foreign proteins invite violent reactions from the protective systems of the host. If foreign proteins enter the body systems and are not quickly eliminated, they can destroy the host. Therefore, the host defense system has to generate a series of responses to eradicate it. The paternal immunological component of the fetus is such a foreign protein. It is not treated any differently by the maternal immune systems. The latter tries all its might to eliminate and destroy the alien. However, miraculously it may seem the fetus allograft survives.

One of the significant roles that are played by a series of actors in this phenomenon is the one that is played by the syncytiotrophoblast. As it is well known, these syncytiotrophoblasts are very specialized cells. The cells of cytotrophoblasts merge or fuse with each other to form the syncytiotrophoblasts. Syncytiotrophoblasts have the capacity to shield the fetus from the maternal onslaught. Syncytiotrophoblasts are immunologically very efficient. They can physically resist destruction by the maternal immune responses. Not only this, the syncytiotrophoblasts have an incredible capacity to protect the fetal system and make it grow. These responses can serve as valuable lessons for transplant scientists.

The biggest bugbear of transplant science is rejection. Preventing this rejection is a big challenge for these scientists. It is therefore proposed that if the transplant scientists can create artificial syncytiotrophoblasts system, the entire rejection phenomenon can be relegated to history. An efficient artificial syncytiotrophoblasts system will protect the graft (in transplant sciences a nonallograft). Just as in the reproductive system, the fetal allograft is allowed to survive and even protected by the host (mother) due to syncytiotrophoblasts, on the same lines as the host system will at the least ignore and not eliminate the graft.

Immune diversity between the mother and fetus is critical. The fetus is expected to be immunologically diverse from the mother because of the component it receives from the father. If the fetus is immunologically similar to the mother, the mother will eliminate it. It seems the syncytiotrophoblasts are programmed to protect only immunologically diverse grafts. If the fetus is immunologically distinct from the mother, it will be protected, nurtured, and made to grow. If it is similar to the mother, it will be eliminated.

Syncytiotrophoblasts sense the immunologically different entity of the fetus and mount a protective response. Understandably this immune differentiation of the fetus has its roots in the father. If one step is traced behind one can understand that if the father is immunologically different from the mother the fetus will also be different. If the father and therefore the fetus are immunologically different, the syncytiotrophoblasts will mount a successful protective response. As a corollary, if the mother and the father are immunologically similar the syncytiotrophoblasts will be rendered hypoefficient. They will then fail to mount a protective response and thereby create an elimination of the fetus. This phenomenon explains the immune rejection in reproduction leading to the clinical entity of fetal demise.

What is Spontaneous Resolution?

In clinical practice, one sees the reality of spontaneous resolutions in subjects with recurrent spontaneous miscarriages. It is most pronounced in whom once the fetal heart activity is demonstrated and then lost. These are usually immunological losses. There is a need to explain spontaneous resolution at this stage. Spontaneous resolution is the happening in which the mother who was repeatedly rejecting the fetal allograft just starts tolerating it after a series of immunological losses. Spontaneous resolution is also attributable to the maternal immune system learning to tolerate the fetus. Vaccination science can help to understanding this phenomenon of immune tolerance better.

In vaccination science, it is a well-known fact that the first dose generates an attenuated response and needs a booster dose for a complete protective response. In the same way, it is possible that the maternal system too learns to tolerate the fetal allograft efficiently in subsequent pregnancies. This learning results in a favorable outcome after failures due to obstetric vasculopathies. This vaccination model as it can be called, may be working in some subjects showing a spontaneous resolution.

Nevertheless, in clinical practice, it also happens that a subject may have a spontaneous and total resolution in third or fourth pregnancy but again some manifestation of an adverse obstetric outcome in fifth or sixth pregnancy. In one of our studies, we found that on long-term follow-up of subjects with PE remote from term, 59.8% developed PE in next pregnancy, and 24.4% developed PE of a severe type. Fetal outcome was consistently poor. There was a high risk for fetal demise and IUGR. These subjects had very high chances of chronic hypertension.[28]

So why is it that some subjects show adverse obstetric outcomes in spite of a successful pregnancy (spontaneous resolution)? The only possible explanation is that in some subjects the requirement of the booster is repeated. Thus, after a successful pregnancy outcome due to the maternal system entirely tolerating that pregnancy again the system slips back to a nonprotection mode and needs one or more pregnancies to evince one more protective response. In vaccination, declining levels of immune responsiveness are time-based. But in human pregnancies with immunological failures, it is not time-based. It means that time between the occurrence of a successful pregnancy outcome and the next pregnancy which fails is not important. In vaccination it is important. It is only on this time factor that booster doses and timings are decided. It, therefore, seems that the vaccination model seems right to understand how maternal systems may learn to tolerate a fetal allograft. Accepted, that it is not entirely applicable in reproductive immunology, this model, however, helps to understand the process better.

At the same time, the event of spontaneous resolution is attributed to the generation of the efficient syncytiotrophoblasts system. In subjects who show an obstetric vasculopathy after a spontaneous resolution, it seems that the key lies in the generation of proficient syncytiotrophoblasts. With every pregnancy, there is a generation of new syncytiotrophoblasts. Learning from the vaccination model, the maternal system it seems may influence in generating an efficient syncytiotrophoblast system once the threshold has been crossed. In such subjects, there is no recurrence of obstetric vasculopathies. But in those subjects in whom there is a recurrence, the maternal system has a limited influence or no influence to cause generation of efficient syncytiotrophoblasts. In them, obstetric vasculopathies recur even after one successful live birth. In which subject this would occur is not predictable. To what extent does the paternal component of the fetus influences, this is also not known.

However, one fact gets solidly crystallized. The syncytiotrophoblasts have a critical role in protecting the conceptus from rejection. Also, they have a privileged status enabling them to generate a miracle of paradox.

THE MIRACLE OF PARADOX

Leads to Transplant Scientists

Any miracle if at all it occurs is intriguing and magnificent. Such a paradox is happening continuously in this process of host-graft interaction. A mother readily tolerates, nourishes, and makes the fetus grow. However, the mother rejects an implant if the donor of the implant is the father of her child. The fetus (child) has two immunological contributions. One is from the mother that is innate to the maternal system. The other component is received from the father. This paternal component is alien to the maternal system. Why then does the mother reject the kidney donated by the father and tolerate the fetus allograft provided by him? Interestingly the physical size of the kidney may be just 1% of the full grown mature fetus still the 100th time smaller kidney gets rejected coming from the incompatible father, but the fetus coming from him is nourished and nurtured. This situation is paradoxical. It becomes further intriguing and surprising as one examines this phenomenon in still further depth.

When the MHC antigens on the mother and the father were studied, it was found that more sharing of these antigens better the possibility of the mother accepting the father's kidney. On the other hand more the sharing of the antigens poorer the chances of the fetus being tolerated. In other words, if the father is immunologically similar to the mother his kidney (or to that matter most other organs) get accepted in the maternal milieu. He is called a compatible donor. However, the fetus bearing the immunological contribution from the same compatible father has a much larger chance to get rejected. If there is an HLA sharing (MHC similarity) the fetus fails to protect itself and the mother fails to nurture the pregnancy. If there is an MHC sharing between the mother and the father, the fetus gets rejected but not the father's organs. On the flip side if they are immunologically diverse their organs get rejected but not their fetus.

LABORATORY EVALUATION

Judgment during pregnancy is tricky as several symptoms and signs also occur in healthy pregnant women. Women with two or more than two spontaneous embryonic/fetal demise especially after the cardiac activity is seen should be screened for APA. It is not necessary to wait for three losses. The suspicion that this may not be cost effective and therefore one should wait for three losses has been summarily disproved.[29] Women with a history of deep vein thrombosis or strong family history of thromboembolism should also be so tested.[30] About 50% of such women will be found to have a thrombophilic defect. The components of thrombophilia panel are:
- Anticardiolipin antibody
- Lupus anticoagulant
- Protein C levels
- Protein S levels
- Antithrombin III levels
- Serum Hcy levels
- Prothrombin 20210 A variant
- Factor V Leiden

Some recommendations do recommend repeating the test. However, in our clinical practice, we do not repeat this test if it is negative or is positive and there is a strong history to support the result.

TREATMENT

Admittedly the treatment of APA syndrome (the autoimmune cause) remains the treatment of effects. It is now a well-known fact that APA syndrome is a result of a decidual vasculopathy. The treatment mainstay is, therefore, aspirin + heparin. Several studies have examined the use of these throughout pregnancy and have demonstrated improved fetal outcomes.[30,31] We have abandoned the use of prednisolone with aspirin for treatment of our positive APA subjects.

Corticosteroids in Recurrent Miscarriage

Some stray studies have claimed that prednisolone administration may improve pregnancy outcomes in women with idiopathic recurrent miscarriage.[32] The effect of prednisolone therapy for some women with recurrent miscarriage may be due to altered endometrial angiogenic growth factor expression and reduced blood vessel maturation.[33] There is ongoing interest in immunosuppressant corticosteroid drugs such as prednisolone to treat infertility in women with repeated in vitro fertilization (IVF) failure and recurrent miscarriage. The rationale draws on the pervasive but flawed view that immune activation is inconsistent with normal pregnancy. It ignores clear evidence that controlled inflammation and activation of the immune response is essential for embryo implantation. Usually, the immune response actively promotes reproductive success by facilitating endometrial receptivity and tolerance of the foreign embryo, and promoting vascular adaptation to support placental morphogenesis. The periconception immune response also establishes developmental trajectories that can impact on fetal growth and gestational age at birth.[34] While women with specific clinical conditions may benefit from the anti-inflammatory and immune-deviating actions of prednisolone and related drugs, it is incorrect to assume a "one-size-fits-all" approach. Better diagnostics and more preclinical studies are essential to define patient groups, build evidence for efficacy, and fine-tune treatments so as not to inhibit necessary actions of immune cells. We argue that unless overt immune pathology is evident, utilization of corticosteroids is not warranted and may be harmful.[34] Studies on regimens using aspirin and prednisolone suggest that complications connected to prednisolone use outweigh the benefits and thus we do not use it anymore.[31]

We follow the following protocol: For all subjects, we give aspirin in a dose of 1.2 mg/kg/day as soon as pregnancy is diagnosed, continue this until 30 weeks, and induce at 37 weeks. We add heparin in a dose of 5,000 IC subcutaneous (SC) daily in the following indications:

- In subjects who test high positive (Table 4.1)
- In subjects who test positive for both lupus and ACA and
- Those subjects who even if low positive have been refractory to only aspirin in previous pregnancy. Heparin too is given up to 36 weeks. We stop a week before induction and induce labor thereafter.

Table 4.1: Interpretation of APA results.

Negative	<10 GPL units
Low positive	10–20 GPL units
Moderate positive	20–100 GPL units
Strong positive	>100 GPL units

Frequently Asked Questions on Heparin

1. **Which heparin—low-molecular weight (fractionated) or regular?**
   Answer: It does not matter. Our results have shown that either molecule does not matter. However, in those subjects on regular heparin, every 3 weeks prothrombin time (PT) and activated partial thromboplastin time (APTT) need to be investigated. If these are increased by more than double the controls, there is a need to stop heparin for a week. The test is to be repeated after that and heparin is restored. Test results usually come to the acceptable band during this period.

2. **What happens if the subject goes into labor or needs to be induced before discontinuing aspirin/heparin?**
   Answer: The fear of bleeding is over blown. It is a platelet bleed. Thus, the bleeding will be diffuse. It will never be unmanageable. Also, this being a platelet bleed, the obstetrician will be needed to apply the hemostatic stitches tighter than usual. This principle holds true even in a cesarean section.
3. **What about the side effect of heparin?**
   Answer: The side effects of heparin in this low-dose regimen are hardly any. Undoubtedly the side effects if any, would be predominantly with the regular (or high-molecular weight) heparin and less with the low-molecular weight preparation. However, the apprehension of osteopenia has been found to be over blown and not found in these subjects. This could be due to low doses as well as the short duration for which we give heparin.
4. **Can we discontinue heparin earlier?**
   Answer: In subjects in whom the pregnancy is progressing satisfactorily and color Doppler parameters are robust, if the uterine artery notching does not occur at or around 20 weeks of trophoblastic invasion is now well handled. In these subjects, we do stop heparin at 28 weeks. However, even in these subjects, we continue low-dose aspirin till term, as in any other subject with APA.

Relevant Observations

- *Remarks on the management of subjects with clinical features of autoimmune losses but testing negative:* These are obviously tricky situations. There are many autoantibodies in circulation which are still within the realms of laboratory research. They are not available for commercial testing in these subjects. Therefore, the order of the day is—if a clinician has reasons to believe that these are necessarily autoimmune losses then he can institute the office said protocol of aspirin or aspirin plus heparin case as the subject demand.
- *Remarks on current understanding of immune potentiation therapy for alloimmune losses:* The treatment regimens

described in under immune potentiating therapy (husband/donor leukocyte transfusions, etc.) have been proved to be of no use. In fact, they can even endanger the life of the subject and should, therefore, be discontinued. Although there is a clear scientific rationale that modulating the maternal immune system could benefit recurrent miscarriage, only a few studies suggest possible beneficial effects of immune modulators as a therapy for recurrent miscarriage. More research is needed to find efficient and safe maternal immune modulators for reproductive pathologies as recurrent miscarriage. Moreover, the possible side effects and neonatal immune function are mostly unknown, and its elucidation is crucial before any possible therapeutic strategies could be clinically implemented.[35]

- *Remarks on different combination with aspirin alone or aspirin plus heparin therapy:* Combinations of immunoglobulins, prednisolone, and like with aspirin alone or in combination with heparin have now been given up. This giving-up is either due to their lack of effectiveness in improving pregnancy outcome or due to a poor risk–benefit ratio.
- *Progesterones:* Use of progesterone especially its compound dehydroprogesterone has been forwarded as immune modulators. Many arguments have come for or against this. The order of the day is in subjects with alloimmune losses where no good therapy is currently available for these agents that may hold promise.
- *Immunoglobulin:* Again this is a gray area in the management of subjects with immunological losses. Their prohibitive cost was considered to be an impediment to widespread use for subjects with immunological recurrent pregnancy losses. Heparin and aspirin are successful in the treatment of elevated APA among women with recurrent miscarriage but not with recurrent implantation failure. Intravenous immunoglobulin (IVIg) has been successful in the treatment of recurrent miscarriage and recurrent implantation failure among women with elevated APA and/or NK cell activity. When the pregnancy outcomes of women with a history of reproductive failure and elevated NK cell

cytotoxicity treated with intralipid were compared with women treated with IVIg, no differences were seen.[36] Immunotherapy for the treatment of reproductive failure enhances live birth but only in those women displaying abnormal immunologic risk factors.[35] As of now, these are of limited use and at best empirical.

- *Sildenafil:* Recently some interest has developed in the use of sildenafil in the management of recurrent miscarriages. It seems favorable results to sildenafil treatment that can be found in subjects with immunological causes of recurrent miscarriages. Positive results of sildenafil treatment are closely connected with its immunomodulatory effects. Sildenafil is believed by these research scientists to be influencing angiogenesis, platelet activation, the proliferation of regulatory T cells, and production of proinflammatory cytokines and autoantibodies.[37] However, sildenafil action in humans and animals appear to be different. In one study, combined sildenafil + heparin therapy was found to be superior to either treatment alone in most analyses. The known safety of sildenafil and heparin in human pregnancy suggests that use of these combined agents may be of value for treatment of patients with impending pregnancy loss or prophylactically in women with a history of recurrent miscarriages.[38] As of now, sildenafil use in recurrent miscarriages seems to be empirical. Further studies will be needed to have a final word on this matter.

SUGGESTED READING

- Immunology of Obstetric Vasculopathy in the book Obstetric Vasculopathies, 1st edition, page 32, Jaypee Brothers Medical Publishers (P) Ltd, New Delhi, 2013 from which this chapter draws on many points and is duly acknowledged.

REFERENCES

1. Sztenc S. Hyperhomocysteinemia and pregnancy complications. Ginekol Pol. 2004;75(4):317-25.
2. Kayaaltı Z, Tekin D, Aliyev V, et al. Effects of the interleukin-6 (IL-6) polymorphism on toxic metal and trace element levels in placental tissues. Sci Total Environ. 2011;409(23):4929-33.

3. Shimada S, Iwabuchi K, Watano K, et al. Expression of allograft inflammatory factor-1 in mouse uterus and poly(I:C)-induced fetal resorption. Am J Reprod Immunol. 2003;50(1):104-12.
4. Marco-Jiménez F, Naturil-Alfonso C, Jiménez-Trigos E, et al. Influence of zona pellucida thickness on fertilization, embryo implantation and birth. Anim Reprod Sci. 2012;132(1-2):96-100.
5. Bell SC, Billington WD. Humoral immune responses in murine pregnancy. III. Relationship between anti-paternal alloantibody levels in maternal serum, placenta and fetus. J Reprod Immunol. 1983;5(5):299-310.
6. Schulz LC, Roberts RM. Dynamic changes in leptin distribution in the progression from ovum to blastocyst of the pre-implantation mouse embryo. Reproduction. 2011;141(6):767-77.
7. Woodruff MF, Anderson NF. The effect of lymphocyte depletion by thoracic duct fistula and administration of antilymphocytic serum on the survival of skin homografts in rats. Ann N Y Acad Sci. 1964;120:119-28.
8. Boyon C, Collinet P, Boulanger L, et al. Fetal microchimerism: benevolence or malevolence for the mother? Eur J Obstet Gynecol Reprod Biol. 2011;158(2):148-52.
9. Brierley J, Clark DA. Characterization of hormone-dependent suppressor cells in the uterus of mated and pseudopregnant mice. J Reprod Immunol. 1987;10(3):201-17.
10. Daya S, Clark DA, Devlin C, et al. Preliminary characterization of two types of suppressor cells in the human uterus. Fertil Steril. 1985;44(6):778-85.
11. Clark DA, Falbo M, Rowley RB, et al. Active suppression of host-vs graft reaction in pregnant mice. IX. Soluble suppressor activity obtained from allopregnant mouse decidua that blocks the cytolytic effector response to IL-2 is related to transforming growth factor-beta. J Immunol. 1988;141(11):3833-40.
12. Tsunawaki S, Sporn M, Ding A, et al. Deactivation of macrophages by transforming growth factor-beta. Nature. 1988;334(6179):260-2.
13. McIntyre JA, McConnachie PR, Taylor CG, et al. Clinical, immunologic, and genetic definitions of primary and secondary recurrent spontaneous abortions. Fertil Steril. 1984;42(6):849-55.
14. Milasinović L, Bulatović S, Ilić D, et al. Adaptation of the immune system as a response to pregnancy. Med Pregl. 2002;55(7-8):305-8.
15. Clark DA. The immunology of recurrent abortion. In: Bonnar J (Ed). Recent Advances in Obstetrics and Gynecology. New York: Churchill Livingstone; 1990. pp. 25-42.
16. Check JH, Katsoff B, Summers-Chase D, et al. A case report supporting the concept that some women have a predisposition for

maternal meiosis errors resulting in digyny. Clin Exp Obstet Gynecol. 2009;36(2):133-4.
17. Choe JK, Check JH, Chern R. Septoplasty allows successful delivery in a primary aborter with six previous first trimester miscarriages. Clin Exp Obstet Gynecol. 2009;36(1):15-6.
18. Papadakis E, Banti A, Kioumi A. Women's Issues in Antiphospholipid Syndrome. Isr Med Assoc J. 2016;18(9):524-9.
19. Miyakis S, Lockshin MD, Atsumi T, et al. International consensus statement on an update of the classification criteria for definite antiphospholipid syndrome (APS). J Thromb Haemost. 2006;4(2):295-306.
20. Matsuura E, Igarashi Y, Fujimoto M, et al. Anticardiolipin cofactor(s) and differential diagnosis of autoimmune disease. Lancet. 1990;336(8708):177-8.
21. McNeil HP, Simpson RJ, Chesterman CN, et al. Anti-phospholipid antibodies are directed against a complex antigen that includes a lipid-binding inhibitor of coagulation: beta 2-glycoprotein I (apolipoprotein H). Proc Natl Acad Sci USA. 1990;87(11):4120-4.
22. Desai P. RSA: current concepts. Indian J Clin Pract. 1992;3(6):13-5.
23. do Prado AD, Piovesan DM, Staub HL, et al. Association of anticardiolipin antibodies with preeclampsia: a systematic review and meta-analysis. Obstet Gynecol. 2010;116(6):1433-43.
24. Infante-Rivard C, David M, Gauthier R, et al. Lupus anticoagulants, anticardiolipin antibodies, and fetal loss. A case-control study. N Engl J Med. 1991;325(15):1063-6.
25. Baroni G, Banzato A, Bison E, et al. The role of platelets in antiphospholipid syndrome. Platelets. 2017:1-5. [Epub ahead of print]
26. Lazzarin N, Vaquero E, Exacoustos C, et al. Midluteal phase Doppler assessment of uterine artery blood flow in nonpregnant women having a history of recurrent spontaneous abortions: correlation to different etiologies. Fertil Steril. 2007;87(6):1383-7.
27. Bello SM, Millo H, Rajebhosale M, et al. Catenin-dependent cadherin function drives divisional segregation of spinal motor neurons. J Neurosci. 2012;32(2):490-505.
28. Desai P, Chandrasekhar G, Udvani HH, et al. Preeclampsia of early onset. J Obstet Gynecol India. 1988;38(5):548.
29. Desai P, Desai M. To what extent is repeat testing necessary for diagnosis of APA syndrome? J Obstet Gynecol India. 1998;48(4):48.
30. Desai P, Desai M, Modi D. Recurrent spontaneous abortion of immunological cause. A case for workup after 2 losses. J Obstet Gynecol India. 1997;47:303.
31. Backos M, Rai R, Baxter N, et al. Pregnancy complications in women with recurrent miscarriage associated with antiphospholipid

antibodies treated with low dose aspirin and heparin. Br J Obstet Gynaecol. 1999;106(2):102-7.
32. Lash GE, Bulmer JN, Innes BA, et al. Prednisolone treatment reduces endometrial spiral artery development in women with recurrent miscarriage. Angiogenesis. 2011;14(4):523-32.
33. Dan S, Wei W, Yichao S, et al. Effect of Prednisolone Administration on Patients with Unexplained Recurrent Miscarriage and in Routine Intracytoplasmic Sperm Injection: A Meta-Analysis. Am J Reprod Immunol. 2015;74(1):89-97.
34. Robertson SA, Jin M, Yu D, et al. Corticosteroid therapy in assisted reproduction—immune suppression is a faulty premise. Hum Reprod. 2016;31(10):2164-73.
35. Prins JR, Kieffer TE, Scherjon SA. Immunomodulators to treat recurrent miscarriage. Eur J Obstet Gynecol Reprod Biol. 2014;181:334-7.
36. Coulam CB, Acacio B. Does immunotherapy for treatment of reproductive failure enhance live births? Am J Reprod Immunol. 2012; 67(4):296-304.
37. Kniotek M, Boguska A. Sildenafil Can Affect Innate and Adaptive Immune System in Both Experimental Animals and Patients. J Immunol Res. 2017;2017:4541958.
38. Luna RL, Nunes AK, Oliveira AG, et al. Sildenafil (Viagra) blocks inflammatory injury in LPS-induced mouse abortion: A potential prophylactic treatment against acute pregnancy loss? Placenta. 2015;36(10):1122-9.

Chapter 5

Genetics of Recurrent Miscarriages and Other Pregnancy Losses

Sharad Gogate

INTRODUCTION

It has been reported that the reproductive loss is much more in *Homo sapiens* than any other species. It is postulated that this high pregnancy wastage is an evolutional measure to keep the human litter size relatively small to permit a long and undistracted rearing time for the newborn. The genetic factors associated with this problem will be considered in this chapter.

ETIOLOGY

Many miscarriages in human beings are due to chromosomal aneuploidies and other chromosomal abnormalities. As many as 70% conceptuses do not survive, of which more than 50% are lost before implantation. Also, 10-20% clinically recognized pregnancies and 2-5% end as perinatal losses.[1,2] With the use of molecular testing like genomic hybridization and microarray, more than 65-70% products of conception (POC) of 1st trimester pregnancy losses show chromosomal anomalies. Higher incidence of chromosomal abnormalities in the gametes is one of the main reasons for this. Oocytes and sperms show aneuploidies in 18-19% and 3-5%, respectively. As a result, 1 in 13 conceptions show chromosomal anomalies.[3] The genetic etiology in various groups of pregnancy losses has been shown in Box 5.1.

> **Box 5.1:** Various etiologies of genetic factors in pregnancy loss.
> - Structural chromosomal anomalies in either partner
> - Chromosomal anomalies in oocyte
> - Chromosomal anomalies in spermatozoa
> - Postfertilization chromosomal anomalies
> - Mosaicism.

Chromosomal Anomalies in Parents

Parents with structural chromosomal anomalies can be fertile and can produce abnormal gametes; it has been shown that one-third of the progeny of mothers with trisomy 21 will also have trisomy. Similarly parents with balanced structural anomalies like Robertsonian translocation, reciprocal translocations, and inversions have aneuploid gametes.[4] Other genetic defects seen in partners are microdeletion of Y-chromosome, cystic fibrosis transmembrane conductance regulator (CFTR) gene mutations on chromosome 7, and androgen receptor gene defect in unexplained in vitro fertilization (IVF) failures. Apparently balanced translocations can become unbalanced during the gametogenesis due to the pairing of deoxyribonucleic acid (DNA) sister chromatid segment during first meiotic division.

Abnormal Oogenesis

Abnormal oogenesis is the most common reason for a majority of the chromosomal aneuploidies; it is because of meiotic errors in the first meiotic division. Less than optimum recombination between sister chromatids, nondisjunction of two sister chromatids, anaphase lag in one of the sister chromatids as well as preseparation of the sister chromatids are the likely mechanisms.[5] The probable reason of the higher abnormalities in oocytes is the fact that the first meiotic division of oocyte starts in fetal life and is completed only after puberty. Various studies have reported widely differing rates of 5–65% with mean somewhere at 23%. These abnormal oocytes can get fertilized resulting in chromosomal abnormalities in the conceptus leading to pregnancy loss. It has been postulated that low levels of 5,10-methylenetetrahydrofolate reductase (MTHFR) gene activity as a high-risk factor for neural tube defect (NTD) as well as Down syndrome.[6] This gene is necessary for methylation of DNA molecule as well as the spindle function by providing methyl groups at the time of meiotic division of the oocyte. So, folic acid supplementation may have some protective role in the prevention of Down syndrome as well as NTD.

Abnormal Spermatogenesis

It has been investigated by many workers, and the incidence varies between 8% and 10%, two-thirds of them show structural abnormalities while one-third shows aneuploidies.

Syngamy

Errors in fertilization are called syngamy, exclusion of female pronucleus and duplication of the male pronucleus results in androgenic syngamy as seen in complete hydatidiform mole. In contrast, there can be a duplication of either male or female pronucleus resulting in triploidy (69 chromosomes). If the male pronucleus duplicates then it results in partial hydatidiform mole (PHM), while duplication of female pronucleus results in triploidy, which can be born with various major malformations. Tetraploidy (96 XXXX/96 XXYY) arises because of failure of cytokinesis; it can be seen more commonly in amniotic fluid, though true embryonic tetraploidy is very rare. It rarely progresses beyond 2-3 weeks. It can be associated with residual trophoblastic disease, requires follow-up.[7]

Postzygotic abnormalities in chromosomes occur due to mitotic errors in early stages of embryonic development resulting in mosaicism (more than one cell line present in the conceptus). Its impact will depend on the stage at which the error develops. Many structural abnormalities like translocation, deletions, and inversion can develop in the postzygotic mitotic divisions. These will result in pregnancy loss or structural/functional anomalies.

Uniparental disomy can result from loss of either maternal or paternal sister chromatid during cell division by nondisjunction or anaphase lag with duplication of the remaining sister chromatid during DNA synthesis. As a result, the chromosome contains only maternal/paternal chromatid. This phenomenon is seen in the placental tissues with resultant growth restriction and stillbirths.

The role of single genes/polygenic/multifactorial factors as the cause of repeated pregnancy losses. Single gene mutations leading to abnormal embryonic development (placental and cardiac lesions) and skewed X-chromosomal inactivation seen in more women with recurrent pregnancy losses indicate such possibility.[8]

Chimerism

It is the presence of, in one individual, of two or more cell lines derived from more than one zygote or individuals. Colonization of maternal cells in the fetus by transplacental route and crossover of cells from monochorionic twins are the likely mechanisms.

Teratogens and Environmental Factors

There can be other causes for chromosomal abnormalities like exposure to ionizing radiation, X-rays, chemotherapeutic drugs as well as other teratogens which results in chromosomal breakages, recombination with resultant loss of pregnancy.

Reactive Oxygen Species

Reactive oxygen species (ROS) are the product of mitochondrial energy generation systems, hence are being produced all the time. These include superoxide anion radical (O_2^-), hydroxyl radical (-OH), nitric oxide, hydrogen peroxide (H_2O_2), and peroxynitrite ($ONOO^-$). All these have an extra electron and can damage to cellular proteins, lipids, and DNA. This happening results in loss of enzyme activity, alteration of cell membranes and damage lesions, and oxidative mutagenesis.[9]

Placenta, embryonic tissues have high mitochondrial activity and produce elevated levels of ROS. Aerobic organisms are protected from ROS damage by efficient enzyme systems as well as antioxidant molecules like cysteine, methionine, carotenoids, selenium, vitamin E, C, etc. While physiological levels of ROS play an important role in the reproductive process as well as embryogenesis, high levels of ROS can have an adverse impact. It can lead to embryopathies, embryonic death, miscarriages, fetal growth restriction, intrauterine growth restriction (IUGR), etc. So far there is no conclusive evidence to suggest a therapeutic use of antioxidants in recurrent pregnancy loss (RPL) cases has any beneficial effect.

Implantation Failure/Very Early Miscarriages

Implantation failure is when the beta human chorionic gonadotropin (hCG) comes positive, but there is no evidence of pregnancy on ultrasonography (USG) along with falling titer of the hormone. This finding is the most frustrating event in the assisted reproductive technology (ART) program and brings down the success rate. The rate of chromosomally abnormal is approximately 40% which includes abnormal chromosomes in oocytes, spermatozoa, and postfertilization chromosomal abnormalities.[10] There is a selection bias against these abnormal embryos at and soon after implantation thus leading to very early miscarriages as well.

BLIGHTED OVUM AND MISSED ABORTION

These are the two most common ways of repeated pregnancy loss seen in the 1st trimester. It has been observed that around 15–20% pregnancies are lost in this manner. In a large multicentric study of 9,113 spontaneous miscarriages, 4,206 (43%) showed chromosomal abnormalities. The types of the abnormalities are shown in Table 5.1[11]

In a similar large study done by Centre for Genetic Health Care, Mumbai similar pattern of chromosomal anomalies were encountered in products of conceptions and have been tabulated in Table 5.2. Different chromosomal anomalies detected, in the same study, from fetal tissue sampling are also shown in Figure 5.1.

Stillbirth and Neonatal Deaths

Stillbirth is defined as the birth of a dead fetus during late 2nd and 3rd trimesters of pregnancy. Neonatal death is defined as death

Table 5.1: Various chromosomal abnormalities seen in abortuses.[12]

Autosomal trisomy	2,097	50%
45,X	776	18%
Triploid/euploid/aneuploidy	650	15%
Tetraploid/aneuploid/euploid	227	5%
Structural	104	4%
Mosaics	155	4%
Trisomy: Double/triple	82	2%
Other	27	1%
Sex chromosome trisomy	26	<1%
Autosomal monosomy	6	<1%
Total	4,206	100%

Table 5.2: Incidence of structural incidence of chromosomal anomalies in abortuses.[13]

CGHS data (2001–2005)				
Number of cases	Normal karyotype	Abnormal karyotype	Culture failure	FISH done in
2,700	1,585	784 (29.04%)	331	60
Percentage of various chromosomal abnormalities				
Type of abnormality		Number of cases		Percentage (%)
Monosomy "X"		365		13.51
Trisomy		194		7.18
Double trisomy		10		0.37
Triploidy		165		6.11
Tetraploidy		10		0.37
Mosaic		15		0.55
Rearrangements		5		0.18
Others		20		0.74

(Center for Genetic Health Care, Mumbai; FISH: fluorescence in situ hybridization)

occurring within 4 weeks of birth. The etiology of stillbirths is very varied and ill determined in a significant percentage of cases. A genetic cause was found in 11.9% of macerated stillbirths, 4.2% of

Genetics of Recurrent Miscarriages and Other Pregnancy Losses

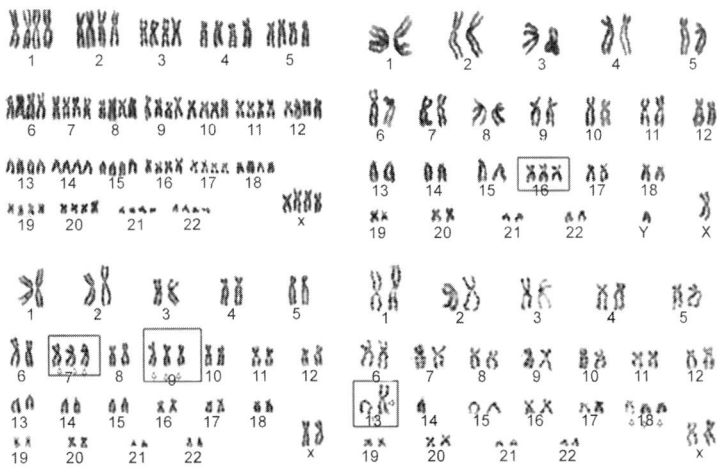

Fig. 5.1: Various types of chromosomal rearrangements.

Table 5.3: Frequency of chromosomal anomalies in perinatal deaths, according to clinical presentation.

Clinical presentation	Abnormal/total	Percentage (%)
Macerated SB, without malformations	8/79	4.5
Macerated SB, with malformations	14/26	54
Severe, multiple anomalies	57/198	29
Congenital heart disease	4/135	3
Primary CNS malformations	0/160	0
Primary associated disease	3/279	1
Fresh SB, without malformations	0/61	0
Primary anoxia	4/233	2
Total	90/1,271	7.0

(CNS: central nervous system; SB: stillbirth)

nonmacerated stillbirths, and 6.0% of neonatal deaths.[13] In another large collaborative study chromosomal abnormalities in perinatal deaths were evaluated according to clinical presentation.[14-16]

Table 5.3 data shows the need for careful evaluation of all cases of perinatal deaths by clinical examination, fetal autopsy, and genetic investigations like cytogenetic, molecular genetic tests to ascertain the exact etiology.

SYNDROMES

By definition, syndrome means a recognizable pattern of structural anomalies which are known or thought to be causally related to the early embryonic developmental stage. A large number of such syndromes have been documented, and it is necessary for clinicians to be aware of such syndromes. The presumption/diagnosis of a syndrome is made, if there is unbalanced chromosomal abnormality or a history of previously affected sibling in X-linked trait, an affected son in a sister or mother's sister or mildly affected parents or consanguinity (first/second degree) in parents, or teratogenic exposure history.[17]

The incidence of structural chromosomal anomalies as shown by Rooney DE, Czepulkowaski BH has been tabulated in Table 5.4.[18]

Table 5.4: Incidence of structural chromosomal abnormalities.

Type of abnormality	Incidence in prenatal tests (1/1,000)	Incidence at birth (1/1,000)
Extra marker chromosome	0.59	0.63
Balanced reciprocal translocation	1.21	2.0
Balanced Robertsonian translocation	0.74	1.35
Unbalanced Robertsonian translocation	0.13	0.07
Inversion	0.36	0.55
Other unbalanced structural abnormalities	0.26	0.19
Inv(9)(p11q13)	–	8.66

CHROMOSOMAL ABNORMALITIES AND FETAL MALFORMATIONS

The presence of certain fetal anomalies is associated with higher chance of chromosomal defects, thus indicating a need for cytogenetic and molecular genetic evaluation.[19] These abnormalities include:
- *Very high risk of chromosomal anomalies (>30%):* Increased nuchal translucency (>3 mm) or nuchal fold in the 2nd trimester or cystic hygroma with or without hydrops, congenital heart

disease, tracheoesophageal fistula/esophageal atresia, Dandy-Walker malformation, and holoprosencephaly.
- *High risk for chromosomal abnormalities (20-30%):* Symmetric IUGR (early onset) with abnormal amniotic fluid volume and anomalies, microcephaly, duodenal atresia and other gastrointestinal (GI) anomalies, facial cleft, omphalocele, and limb defects.
- *Moderate risk (10-20%):* Hyperechoic bowel, renal anomalies, isolated hydrocephaly/ventriculomegaly, congenital diaphragmatic hernia (if associated with other abnormalities), and oligo/polyhydramnios.
- *Low risk (<10%):* Isolated NTD, clubfoot, choroid plexus cyst, single umbilical artery, pyelectasis, and echogenic cardiac focus.

INVESTIGATIVE WORKUP FOR GENETIC CAUSES OF RECURRENT PREGNANCY LOSS

A suggested outline for evaluation of early pregnancy loss and fetal malformation is shown in Box 5.2.[12]

History

- Maternal medical history of systemic medical disorders like diabetes, cardiovascular, endocrine disorders, ongoing medication, exposure to teratogens, exanthematous infections, etc.
- Family history (on both maternal and paternal sides) of unexplained repeated pregnancy losses, stillbirths, congenital anomalies, cancers, sudden deaths, single gene disorders like hemoglobinopathies, metabolic errors, etc.
- It is also essential to prepare a pedigree chart of the family.
- Previous obstetric history of pregnancy losses, birth defects, stillbirth, prematurity, perinatal deaths, any investigations of genetic testing, or postmortem studies done on the affected child.
- *Evaluation of the present pregnancy:* Pregnancy duration by last menstrual period (LMP), pregnancy duration by dating scan, problems in the 1st trimester, problems in 2nd trimester,

> **Box 5.2:** Evaluation protocol for early fetal loss and malformation.
>
> - *Gather pertinent history:*
>   - General medical, genetic
>   - Obstetric
>   - Occupational, environmental, etc.
>
> - *Pathology protocol:*
>   - Gross examination
>   - Microscopy
>   - Photography
>   - Radiography, other imaging
>
> - *Special studies:*
>   - Chromosomal analysis, deoxyribonucleic acid (DNA) diagnosis, metabolic studies, etc.
>   - Muscle analysis
>   - Electron microscopy
>   - Neuropathology
>   - Infectious diseases
>   - Fibroblast culture (for biochemical studies)
>   - Chemical analysis
>   - Cell bank, DNA library
>
> - *Consultations (as required):*
>   - Medical geneticist
>   - Fetal medicine
>   - Biochemistry
>   - Neuropathology
>   - Infectious diseases
>   - Teratology
>   - Imaging sciences
>   - Others
>
> - Compilation of all reports, final diagnosis
> - Follow-up multispecialty consultation with family and referring physicians.

problems in 3rd trimester, drugs/radiation/teratogens/infections, anomalies on USG, maternal serum screening for Down syndrome, NTD, infection screening, and APL syndrome.

Physical Examination

- *General examination:* Look for any dysmorphic features, endocrine disorders, cardiac, renal, immunological disorders, etc.

- Gynecological examination for any congenital anomalies/injuries.
- Obstetric examination for any local or general complication of pregnancy.
- Examination of male partner.
- Examination of affected members of the family.

Investigations

Autopsy and Other Fetal Pathology Workups

The fetal autopsy and other pathology workup play very vital role in investigations of genetic and other causes of pregnancy losses. These studies help in clinching a final diagnosis of the underlying cause, assist in arriving at proper risk of recurrence, and provide valuable help for preconception counseling and management. Unfortunately, both the managing clinicians and the patient's family fail to grasp the need of this vital investigation, due to various reasons, at the time of termination/delivery of an affected fetus and loose a valuable opportunity.

A fetal autopsy should be done as per a well-developed protocol, which includes noting down of clinical notes, detail history, through physical examination and photography. With an easy availability of mobile phones with digital cameras, it should not be difficult to prepare a photo library. This image collection is particularly useful when the relatives refuse permission for a full autopsy for emotional/religious reasons (virtual autopsy).

The fetal body should be kept in cold storage, and formalin saline should be injected in all body cavities including skull to prevent autolysis. A thorough autopsy has to be done to study internal anatomy and obtain samples for histology, special staining, and other specialized tests like genetic tests, microbiological, and toxicological tests. It is also necessary to set up cell bank and DNA library for preserving tissue samples of rare disorders for future research and therapy as well as preconception evaluation and treatment in subsequent conceptions. Histopathology of products of conception: Routine hematoxylin and eosin (H&E) staining, specialized staining techniques, histochemistry, and electron microscopy can add value to the autopsy workup.

Table 5.5: Histological studies of products of conception. Total number of samples studied 750.

Gestation period	Genetic factor	Infection	Vascular insufficiency	Nonidentifiable
1st trimester	65%	20%	–	15%
2nd trimester	50%	40%	–	10%
3rd trimester	20%	30%	30%	30%

Etiological causes of fetal loss that can be diagnosed by morphology and histopathology include infections, chromosomal defects, and vascular insufficiency. Features that indicate chromosomal anomalies are embryonic growth stunting, empty gestational sac, and ruptured sac without embryo or cord. Microscopic features which are seen include dysmorphic villi, hypovascularity, and trophoblastic inclusions.

Based on these criteria more than 65–70% concordance was observed when cytogenetic analysis was done in cases with histopathology s/o genetic factors.[20] A result of 750 subjects has been tabulated in Table 5.5.

Fetal Tissue Sampling for Genetic Evaluation

Fetal tissue sampling is one of the most important investigations for proper diagnosis and evaluation of genetic causes of pregnancy loss. With rapid advances in imaging modalities like conventional USG, three-dimensional (3D) and four-dimensional (4D) scans, sono-CT, and MRI our ability to study the fetus in health and disease have improved considerably. Improved genetic screening tests, rapid advances in DNA technology is making fast and accurate diagnosis of genetic defects possible. In spite of this progress, direct access to fetal tissues is still required in a significant number of disorders for confirmation of diagnosis and prognostication.

The fetal tissues can be obtained for evaluation at antemortem or postmortem stage, but it is preferable to obtain tissue samples at an antenatal stage to have better preserved, less contaminated, and more targeted samples which will be more easily cultured.

> **Box 5.3:** Fetal tissue sampling techniques.
>
> Preimplantation genetic diagnosis (PGD)
> - Polar body/blastomere biopsy/trophectoderm biopsy
>
> 1st trimester sampling
> - Chorionic villous sampling (CVS), early amniocentesis
>
> 2nd trimester sampling
> - Amniocentesis, late CVS, cordocentesis, and other fetal tissue samplings
>
> Noninvasive sampling
> - Fetal cells in maternal blood
> - Tissue samples obtained during fetal autopsy.

Karyotyping of POC has rather poor results due to nonviability of tissues, maternal cell contamination and overgrowth, and culture failure. With improvements in the tissue culture techniques, use of molecular diagnostic techniques like quantitative fluorescent polymerase chain reaction (QF-PCR), multicolor fluorescence in situ hybridization (M-FISH), molecular karyotyping, comparative genomic hybridization (CGH), etc. successful diagnosis of genetic disorders can be done in postmortem samples as well.

The opinion is divided about routine fetal karyotyping from POC as part of the investigative protocol. Proponents emphasize the benefits of accurate diagnosis, specific, sensitive genetic counseling, and categorization of the risk of recurrence. The opponents feel that there is no conclusive proof of tangible benefits, clinical justification, or psychological benefit by routine fetal karyotyping in POC.[21] Various fetal tissue sampling techniques used are shown in Box 5.3.

There are some problems in performing fetal tissue sampling. The postgraduate training programs do not cover these techniques. As a result, there is a shortage of adequately trained clinicians. Nonavailability of proper imaging equipment, underutilization of existing infrastructure, lack of coordination, and planning between clinic and laboratory also contribute to the difficulties.

It is important to consider following points before undertaking fetal tissue sampling:
- Indication for the sampling procedure
- Appropriate timing for the test

- Risk of recurrence of the disease
- Risk of the procedure, for mother and fetus
- Reliability of the procedure (clinical and laboratory)
- Proper pre- and postprocedure counseling.

Once the fetal tissue sample is collected, it should be checked for quality and quantity transferred in transport medium, supplied by the testing laboratory, before the patient is allowed to go home. The sample should be accompanied by all clinical details, previous investigations, and expected tests to be performed on the sample. In the laboratory various tests like karyotyping, high-resolution banding, molecular diagnostic tests like FISH, PCR, etc. should be performed with strict quality control and standard protocols. The results should be sent with explanatory notes, interpretation of the results, and genetic counseling.

Parental karyotyping: Opinion is divided about the need for parental karyotyping in genetic evaluation. Accepted indications are:

- Suspected/clinically distinct chromosomal syndrome/disorder
- Mental retardation with/without malformations
- Abnormal sexual development
- Unexplained infertility/ART failures
- Previous child with a structural chromosomal abnormality
- Repeated pregnancy losses (>3), unexplained stillbirths
- Exposure to chemotherapeutic agents/radiation

These studies should be done at preconception stage itself to permit proper evaluation and preventive steps. High-resolution banding, molecular cytogenetic techniques like FISH, QF-PCR, and CGH should be done to evaluate single gene disorders, microdeletion syndromes.[21]

GENETIC COUNSELING

Genetic counseling is a crucial aspect of the genetic workup. After all the earlier investigations are done, one has to try and arrive at the final diagnosis. It should be done ideally at the preconception stage itself, and a multispecialty team approach is ideal. A dedicated team comprising of geneticist, fetal medicine expert, pediatrician, pediatric surgeon, imaging specialist, and teratologist and metabolic disorders specialist are needed to handle the complex situations of genetic disorders.

The counseling should address following important aspects:
- Reason for referral
- Detailed history of patient and family (genetically targeted)
- Thorough physical checkup
- Necessary laboratory, imaging, and other investigations
- Preparing pedigree charts
- Evaluation of natural history of the disorder, likely complications
- Estimating the accurate recurrence risk, this can be very difficult task at times
- Measures required include: (1) Incidence of the disorder in general population, (2) Inheritance pattern, (3) Database from other centers, (4) Pedigree charting, (5) Screening tests, and (6) Use of statistical methodologies.

Once the risk of recurrence is understood, we have to try and prevent the same. Various measures towards this aim include:
- Premarital counseling
- Preconception counseling
- Genetic studies in parents and affected members
- *Prenatal diagnosis, management:* Important factors to be considered include: (1) Availability of appropriate test, (2) Reliability, specificity of test, (3) Clinical and laboratory risks of the test, and (4) Risk to benefit ratio (both for mother and fetus).

MANAGEMENT

The management depends to a great extent on the exact cause of the genetic disorder resulting in pregnancy loss and the risk of recurrence. In case the risk of recurrence is low and antenatal diagnosis is available then preconception therapy with folic acid, zinc, and vitamin B12 should be started at least 2 months before conception and continued for the 1st trimester. Usual genetic screening tests like 1st and 2nd trimester maternal serum screening for NTD, Down syndrome along with anomaly scans are indicated. Wherever indicated, fetal tissue sampling and prenatal diagnosis are offered. Intensive monitoring throughout the conception, the birth of the child in a proper healthcare facility, and careful neonatal evaluation by an experienced pediatric geneticist is a must.

With the availability of IVF-embryo transfer (ET) along with preimplantation genetic diagnosis (PGD), in situations with high risk of recurrence only unaffected embryos are implanted. It avoids the trauma of termination of an affected fetus.

When the risk of recurrence is high like in autosomal dominant disorders and Robertsonian type of translocations, use of donor egg or sperm along with ART is offered. In some scenarios, adoption may become more practical and humane alternative, though not that easy to accept.

CONCLUSION

It is true that our genetic blueprint is beyond our control and comprehensively regulates the development, functioning of the human body in health and disease. Contrary to belief, our genetic destiny is not preordained. By implementing multispecialty, holistic, and preventive approach at all stages of life we can make a lot of difference in incidence of repeated pregnancy loss, genetic disorders, their severity, the chances of survival, and quality of life of our patients and their families.

Note: Author of this chapter Dr Sharad Gogate is Director, Surlata Hospital and Fetal Medicine Consultancy Services, Mumbai, India.

REFERENCES

1. Hertig AT, Rock J, Adams EC, et al. Thirty-four fertilized human ova, good, bad and indifferent, recovered from 210 women of known fertility; a study of biologic wastage in early human pregnancy. Pediatrics. 1959;23(1 Part 2):202-11.
2. Leridon H. Human Fertility: Basic Components. Illinois: Chicago University press; 1977.
3. Martin RH, Ko E, Rademaker A. Distribution of aneuploidy in human gametes. Am J Med Genet. 1991;39(3):321-31.
4. Hamerton JL. Tables 5-10. New York: Academic Press; 1971.
5. Delhanty JD. Mechanisms of aneuploidy induction in human oogenesis and early embryogenesis. Cytogenet Genome Res. 2005;111(3-4):237-44.

6. James SJ, Pogribna M, Pobribny IP, et al. Abnormal folate metabolism and mutation in the methylenetetrahydrofolate reductase gene may be maternal risk factors for Down syndrome. Am J Clin Nutr. 1999;70(4):495-501.
7. Simpson JL. Genetics of spontaneous abortions. In: Carp HJ (Ed). Recurrent Pregnancy Loss: Causes, Controversies, and Treatment, 2nd edition. Florida: CRC Press; 2014. pp. 21-33.
8. Regan L, Backos M, Farquharson RG. Pregnancy strategies. In: James DK, Steer PJ, Weiner CP, Gonik B (Eds). High Risk Pregnancy: Management Options, 4th edition. Philadelphia: Elsevier Saunders; 2011. p. 77.
9. Agarwal A, Aziz N, Rizk B. Oxidative Stress and Prenatal Developmental Outcomes: Studies on Women's Health. New York: Humana Press; 2013. pp. 3-7.
10. Plachot M. Chromosomal abnormalities in oocytes. Mol Cell Endocrinol. 2001;183 Suppl 1:S59-63.
11. Martin RH, Spriggs E, Rademaker AW. Multicolor fluorescence in situ hybridization analysis of aneuploidy and diploidy frequencies in 225,846 sperm from 10 normal men. Biol Reprod. 1996;54(2):394-8.
12. Machin GA. Cytogenetic aspects of reproductive loss. In: Reed GB, Claireaux AE, Cockburn F (Eds). Diseases of the Fetus and Newborn. London: Chapman and Hall Medical; 1995. pp. 227-59.
13. Purandarey HM. Genetic Diagnosis in Products of Conception. Mumbai: Centre for Genetic Health Care; 2007.
14. Milunsky A, Benn PA. Prenatal diagnosis of chromosomal abnormalities through amniocentesis. In: Benn PA (Ed). Genetic Disorders and the Fetus, 6th edition. Boston: Boston University; 2010.
15. Sutherland GR, Carter RF, Bauld R, et al. Chromosome studies at the paediatric necropsy. Ann Hum Genet. 1978;42(2):173-81.
16. Sutherland GR, Carter RF. Cytogenetic studies: an essential part of the paediatric necropsy. J Clin Pathol. 1983;36(2):140-2.
17. Angell RR, Sandison A, Bain AD. Chromosomal studies in investigations of stillbirths and perinatal deaths. Arch Dis Child. 1974;49:782-8.
18. Opitz JM, Czeizel A, Evans JA, et al. Nosologic Groupings in Birth Defects. Human Genetics: Proceedings of VIIth International Congress on Human Genetics; 1987. pp. 382-5.
19. Rooney DE, Czepulkowski BH. Human Cytogenetics: Essential Data. New Jersey: John Wiley and Sons; 1994. pp. 1-16.
20. Bieber FR, Driscoll SG. Evaluation of early pregnancy loss. In: Reed GB, Claireaux AE, Cockburn F (Eds). Diseases of the Fetus and Newborn. London: Chapman and Hall Medical; 1995. pp. 175-86.
21. Carp HJ. Should Fetal Karyotype be Performed Routinely in RPL? London: Informa Healthcare; 2008. pp. 35-43.

Chapter 6

Endocrinal Causes of Recurrent Spontaneous Miscarriages

INTRODUCTION

Following implantation, the maintenance of the pregnancy is dependent on a multitude of endocrinological events that will eventually aid in the successful growth and development of the fetus. These events are intricately interwoven with immunological events that have been extensively described in Chapter 4. Although the vast majority of pregnant women have no preexisting endocrine abnormalities, a small number of women can have certain endocrine alterations that could potentially lead to recurrent spontaneous miscarriages. It is estimated that approximately 8–12% of all pregnancy losses are the result of endocrine factors.[1]

During the preimplantation period, stimulated by estrogen and progesterone, the uterus undergoes substantial changes. Progesterone is critically essential for the successful implantation and maintenance of pregnancy. Therefore, disorders of inadequate progesterone secretion by the corpus luteum are likely to affect the outcome of the pregnancy. Adequate luteal phase function is a result of normal follicular development. Any factor that affects follicular development can be reflected in the quality of the consequent luteal phase. Also, hypersecretion of luteinizing hormone (LH) during folliculogenesis has now been proved to hurt both, the fertilization of the ovum and the organization of a healthy early pregnancy.

Luteal phase deficiency, hyperprolactinemia, and polycystic ovarian syndrome (PCOS) are some examples of endocrinal disorders that can disrupt a healthy pregnancy. Several other endocrinological abnormalities such as thyroid disease, hypoparathyroidism, uncontrolled diabetes, and decreased ovarian reserve have been implicated as etiological factors for recurrent spontaneous miscarriages. This article reviews current evidence on the role of endocrinology in recurrent pregnancy miscarriages.

DIABETES AND RECURRENT SPONTANEOUS MISCARRIAGES

Technically diabetes is not a reproductive endocrinopathy. However, its uncontrolled state has been associated with recurrent pregnancy loss. The association between a sporadic miscarriage and stillbirths is proved.[2] However, this association is not so well proved with recurrent spontaneous miscarriages. Subjects with high glycosylated hemoglobin A levels in the 1st trimester are at substantially greater risk of both miscarriage and fetal abnormality.[3,4] It is estimated that early miscarriage rate in well-controlled diabetic women is 15%. This rate may increase to 45% in women with poorly controlled glucose levels. However, screening for occult diabetes mellitus, in asymptomatic women who have normal blood glucose levels presenting with recurrent spontaneous miscarriage in the 1st trimester, seems to have a limited value.[5]

THYROID ABNORMALITIES AND RECURRENT SPONTANEOUS MISCARRIAGES

There is no direct evidence of an association between thyroid dysfunction, and recurrent pregnancy loss.[6,7] Antithyroid antibodies are more commonly found in women with recurrent miscarriage. However, these seem to be a result of a generalized autoimmune aberration rather than a thyroid problem. It is because the results of thyroid function tests in these subjects are consistently found to be normal. Therefore, it is not recommended to screen a subject having a recurrent miscarriage for a thyroid disorder as a routine.[8] In one more study, no significant associations were observed between miscarriage and impaired thyroid function.[9] However, in subjects with other clinical manifestations of thyroid anomalies, the need for treating that anomaly is of course mandatory.

Subclinical hyperthyroidism (SCH) is one more entity which has caught fancy of some research scientists working in this field. Some estimates put the incidence of SCH to about 19% if not more. But it is also wisely concluded that although there was a high prevalence of SCH in the recurrent early pregnancy loss (REPL) cohort, there was no statistically significant difference in the subsequent live-birth rate when comparing women with SCH and euthyroid women, or treated and untreated SCH.[10,11] SCH seems to be overhyped in current clinical practice. Many vague and amorphous associations have been stated between SCH and clinical manifestations. Thankfully, this is one condition where no such connection is proved. This vindicates the stand that there is no need of investigating or treating thyroid disorders in the absence of clinical manifestations.

PROGESTERONE AND RECURRENT SPONTANEOUS MISCARRIAGES

Low Progesterone Levels and Recurrent Miscarriages

The word "progesterone" itself suggests a molecule that is pro— for, gesterone—gestation. This term indicates that progesterone is the hormone that supports pregnancy physiologically. Called the pregnancy hormone, natural progesterone is essential before pregnancy. It has a crucial role in its maintenance based on different mechanisms. These include modulation of maternal immune response and suppression of inflammatory response (the presence of progesterone and its interaction with progesterone receptors at the decidua level appears to play a significant role in the maternal defense strategy). It also includes reduction of uterine contractility (adequate progesterone concentrations in myometrium can counteract prostaglandin stimulatory activity as well as oxytocin). Also, improvement of uteroplacental circulation and luteal phase support (it has been demonstrated that progesterone may promote the invasion of extravillous trophoblasts to the decidua by inhibiting apoptosis of extravillous trophoblasts).[12]

It was about 8 decades ago that studies were published suggesting that a defect in progesterone secretion causes miscarriages.[13]

Progesterone is the critical hormone that converts a proliferative endometrium into a nidable secretory hormone.[14] In early pregnancy, progesterone is released by corpus luteum. It has been successfully shown that lutectomy leads to miscarriage.[15] It has also been shown that in lutectomized subjects, parenteral treatment with progesterone can save the pregnancy.

A very interesting phenomenon relates to the 'implantation window'. It is noteworthy that though the entire endometrium undergoes a secretory change postovulation the implantation takes place only at a point where the implantation window opens. It has now been found that the strongest influence on this phenomenon is progesterone. Under its effect, the implantation window opens early and remains open for a longer time. This further reinforces the role of progesterone in early pregnancy. Results of studies in this regard conclude that natural progesterone treatment in patients with a confirmed hormone deficiency during the luteal phase may not reduce the risk of miscarriage in the overall population of pregnant women, but improves the prognosis compared to the group of women suffering from recurrent miscarriages, thereby reducing the risk to that in the general population.[16]

Luteal Phase Defect and Recurrent Miscarriages

Inadequate progesterone production resulted in an array of clinical disorders including infertility, failed implantation, and early pregnancy loss. Inadequate luteal phase has been reported to occur in 23-60% of patients with recurrent miscarriage.[17,18] Although the literature contains ample studies of luteal phase defect (LPD), there is no reliable technique with which to diagnose inadequate luteal function in conception cycles or early pregnancy. Investigations have focused for the most part on luteal phase progesterone levels and endometrial biopsies in the nonfertile menstrual cycle. Low levels of progesterone in luteal phase are associated with recurrent miscarriage and have been a constant finding together with substantiation of slow endometrial growth. Luteal phase deficiency is more likely to be a result of an abnormal response of the endometrium to progesterone than to a below normal production of progesterone by the corpus luteum. It is with this rationale it is believed that it is superior to treat a malfunctioning endometrium of LPD by artificially stimulating ovulation rather than supplementing progesterone. This debate therefore continues.

PROGESTERONE AND HUMAN CHORIONIC GONADOTROPINS SUPPLEMENTATION IN THE TREATMENT OF RECURRENT SPONTANEOUS MISCARRIAGES

There are lots of controversies that surround progesterone and human chorionic gonadotropin (HCG) supplementation in this treatment. Thankfully, in the light of recent literature, some of these controversies have cleared due to new and better quality evidence. These controversies relate to the agent of choice—HCG or progesterone? If progesterone, then which progesterone and if not progesterone, should the proliferative phase be corrected to get the results. Proliferative phase correction is based on the fact that if the proliferative phase is defective than the luteal phase can be defective. If that be so, can estrogen supplementation help in these cases? It is said that whenever there is a controversy between the "wise", the observers should refrain from taking stands. Therefore, attempts are made here to put before the readers different views. At the same time if and whenever possible, a position will be taken if it does not add to the already turbulent picture.

Human Chorionic Gonadotropin

Theoretically, supplementation of HCG in the luteal phase should fuel progesterone production by the corpus luteum. That is a sound enough rationale for supplementing HCG. Unusual HCG production probably results from a faulty conceptus, in which case HCG therapy would be improper.[19] Amidst this conflicting basis, Cochrane review has taken an interesting stand on this matter. It states that luteal phase support with HCG or progesterone after assisted reproduction results in an increased pregnancy rate. By and large, all recent studies indicate that HCG (5,000 IU twice a week) supplementation may not be superior to progesterone in LPD-related recurrent miscarriages. HCG does not provide better results than progesterone and is associated with a greater risk of ovarian hyperstimulation syndrome (OHSS) when used with gonadotropin-releasing hormone analogs (GnRHa).

Immunological Basis of Using Human Chorionic Gonadotropin[20]

Due to the earlier reasons one low dose of HCG administration and weekly administration, it was perceived that HCG if administered in this way should not produce any results. But in spite of this "low dose," there were studies and experiences in which HCG did produce results even at these schedules and dosages. These results led to exploring the possibility of HCG having effects beyond its biological half-life. The endocrinal (biological) half-life of HCG is indeed 72 hours. Why it is that there are experiences which showed a successful prevention of obstetric vasculopathy even on administration at a weekly duration? The answer lies in the immunological face of HCG.

Every hormone has an endocrinal face and an immunological face. This immune face is what seems to be acting if at all, in the prevention of late 1st trimester and 2nd trimester fetal demise leading to missed abortions. HCG is a master conductor of the immunological orchestra that brings about the immune tolerance in the mother.

Human chorionic gonadotropin oversees and even induces distinct changes in the maternal milieu in such a way that the mother learns to tolerate the foreign immunological protein of the fetus. It either generates changes in the trophoblasts to make them resist the immune rejection of the mother. Alternatively, it may be subduing the immune rejection process. It is also possible that exogenous and endogenous HCG may be doing both.

This understanding brings one closer to the understanding of why lower doses of HCG are effective. Any immunological substance generates its effects much beyond the pharmacological dosage of its administration. The classical example of this is vaccine inoculums. Miniscule doses of vaccine antigens can produce a massive antibody response saving from specific diseases for years. Vaccine inoculums continue to have a protective effect much beyond its presence in the body of the host. Decades after an immunologically active vaccine has been administered, the host gets protected from diseases for which the vaccine was administered. On the same basis, low-dose immunologically active substances can produce effects much more and disproportionate to the amount injected.

It is not to say that HCG is a vaccine. It indeed is not one. But this rationale helps understanding how its low doses can produce effective results much beyond the pharmacological half-life of the hormone administered. Therefore, the immunological half-life of HCG seems to outstrip the endocrinal half-life. It is for this immunological face that HCG is effective at lower doses and that too well beyond the duration of its endocrinal activity.

Dose and Administration

We use HCG in very few subjects for prevention of obstetric vasculopathies. These are mostly refractory subjects in whom fetal demise has occurred in spite of progesterone administration in the past. We also feel that till the time as HCG efficacy is entirely ruled out or committed to science, it should be left to the discretion of the attending clinician if and when he/she wants to administer HCG in clinical practice. As mentioned we administer HCG only in refractory subjects in a dose of 5,000 IU every weekly. This administration is commenced from the diagnosis of pregnancy as early as possible in 1st trimester. We continue HCG till 12 weeks of gestation. It is with a rationale that placenta takes over the function of corpus luteum. Also by this duration the immunological tolerance in whatever form is nearly set in the maternal system.

A latest Cochrane review included five randomized controlled studies, involving 596 women.[21] When comparing the women who were treated with HCG versus placebo or no treatment, these workers found a benefit in using HCG. However, when two of the older studies with weaker methodology were excluded, the evidence of a benefit of using HCG for preventing recurrent spontaneous miscarriages became less apparent. There were no documented adverse effects associated with using HCG. As a result, the authors were unable to make firm recommendations.[21] More good quality studies with larger sample sizes are needed to evaluate the use of HCG compared with other treatments and nonpharmacological strategies, such as early and accessible career contact and support.[21] For clinicians, therefore, the message emerging out of this latest review is that there is no need to change their policy of HCG administration, as of now.

Progesterone

Progesterone appears to be necessary to support an early pregnancy, and it has been used for this purpose for several decades. Its potential role in women with recurrent miscarriage due to luteal phase deficiency has been suggested, but its efficacy has not yet been demonstrated. So as to take a clear stand on the effectiveness of progesterone, it must be assessed through prospective, double-blind, and randomized controlled trials in the light of the results of this meta-analysis.[22]

Progesterone has been administered orally, intramuscularly, and vaginally for more than 5 decades in an attempt to prevent miscarriage in early-to-mid pregnancy. The scientific basis and consistency of results have always been debated. As a result, despite substantial medical use, there is currently inadequate information to allow certain and firm recommendations regarding optimal dose, route, and timing of progesterone supplementation. There is no case to support the routine use of progesterone in the 1st trimester to prevent miscarriage in all subjects in the absence of any known etiological factor. However, one fact is settled. The use of progestational agents during the 1st and 2nd trimester of pregnancy is not associated with adverse effects in mothers.

Which Progesterone and How Much?

In clinical practice natural micronized progesterone 200 mg twice a day vaginally is what is recommended. It may not reduce the risk of miscarriage in the overall population of pregnant women but improves the prognosis.[16]

A recent Cochrane review states that there was evidence, however, that women who have suffered three or more miscarriages may benefit from progestogen during pregnancy. Four trials showed a decrease in miscarriage compared with placebo or no treatment in these women.[23] However, these findings should be interpreted with caution. No differences were found between the route of administration of progestogen (oral, intramuscular, and vaginal). More trials are needed and are under way to further clarify the effects in women with multiple prior miscarriages.[23] For clinicians, therefore, the message on the basis of this latest review is there is no need to change their policy of progesterone administration as of now.

Dydrogesterone

Dydrogesterone has also been evaluated in such cases. Miscarriages were significantly ($p < $ or $= 0.05$) less frequent in the dydrogesterone group (13.4%) than in the control group (29%). There were no differences between the groups concerning pregnancy complications or congenital abnormalities.[24] From this study it seems hormonal support with dydrogesterone can increase the chances of a successful pregnancy in women with a history of recurrent spontaneous miscarriages. In a recently published review by Carp, he has shown a significant reduction of 29% in the odds for miscarriage when dydrogesterone is compared to standard care indicating a real treatment effect. However, all the predictive and confounding factors could not be controlled for, the results of this review.[25]

Cervical Cerclage and Vaginal Progesterone

One of the most common interventions in subjects with recurrent spontaneous miscarriages is cervical cerclage. One of the reasons this is done is to reinforce the incompetent cervix and thereby prevent preterm births (PTBs) in these subjects of recurrent miscarriages. For quite some time now progesterone is forwarded as a replacement to "the invasive" cervical cerclage. Time is ripe enough to find out if progesterone is superior to cervical cerclage in these subjects. One recent study has shown that cervical cerclage had more benefits in the maternal and neonatal outcomes than progesterone therapy for women with an asymptomatic short cervix and prior PTB history, while cervical cerclage and vaginal progesterone therapies showed similar effectiveness for women with an asymptomatic short cervix but without a history of PTB.[12]

LUTEINIZING HORMONE ENDOCRINOPATHY AND RECURRENT SPONTANEOUS MISCARRIAGES

It is well known that the pituitary gland secretes two hormones: (1) LH, and (2) Follicle-stimulating hormone (FSH). In general, LH controls the production of female hormones (estrogen and progesterone) in the ovary, and FSH controls the development of follicles and ovulation. LH and FSH are released in pulses from the pituitary gland in response to stimulation by gonadotropin-releasing hormone (GnRH) from the brain. Specifically, fast GnRH pulses appear to favor LH secretion, and slow GnRH pulses support FSH secretion. The key point is that the pulses of GnRH are slowed by the elevated levels of estrogen and progesterone that occur after ovulation. Studies suggest that this slowing of GnRH allows for later FSH secretion (at the time of menstruation), which normally leads to egg development in the next cycle. These same studies would suggest that if GnRH pulses are not slowed down, subsequent FSH production is diminished.[26] One can, therefore, see that this ability to slow GnRH pulses seems to be quite necessary for subsequent FSH secretion, and therefore subsequent folliculogenesis.

Studies have shown that GnRH secretion in patients with PCOS is relatively fast and that it does not slow down very well in response to estrogen and progesterone. This phenomenon helps to explain why PCOS patients frequently do not ovulate. Women with PCOS often have high levels of LH secretion. Elevated levels of LH contribute to the high levels of androgens (male hormones such as testosterone), and this along with low levels of FSH contributes to the poor follicular development and an inability to ovulate. A lack of ovulation also leads to relative deficiencies of progesterone production by the ovary, which often leads to an absence of menstrual periods.

While many women with PCOS still have LH and FSH still within the 5–20 mIU/mL range, their LH level is often two or three times that of the FSH level. For example, it is typical for women with PCOS to have LH levels of around 18 mIU/mL and FSH levels of around 6 mIU/mL. It should be noted that both levels fall within their range of normalcy of 5–20 mIU/mL. This situation is called an elevated LH to FSH ratio or a ratio of 3:1.[27] This change in the LH to FSH ratio is enough to disrupt ovulation. While this used to be considered an important aspect in diagnosing PCOS, it is now considered less useful in diagnosing PCOS but is still helpful when looking at the overall picture.

It seems, therefore, that in PCOS patients stimulated for in vitro fertilization (IVF) with human menopausal gonadotropin (HMG), follicular phase LH levels have an adverse effect on follicle and oocyte numbers as well as on oocyte quality. Moreover, an inappropriately raised LH appears to have a deleterious effect on the pregnancy outcome by being associated with a greater possibility of miscarriage. On the other hand, the administration of GnRHa in the long desensitization protocol seems to reverse the detrimental effect of increased LH concentrations on follicular and oocyte development, whereas the beneficial effect on oocyte maturity, although significant, appears to be less profound. Furthermore, GnRHa administration is associated with a decreased risk of early miscarriage.

Data also suggests that the hypersecretion of LH rather than the occurrence of PCO are more solidly connected with a meager reproductive result. In a big series of PCO, women with high LH concentrations had a significantly high prevalence of infertility than women with normal LH levels.[26] In a study, it was shown that the occurrence of PCO did not foretell miscarriage, but the patients who miscarried had higher levels of free testosterone than recurrent spontaneous abortion (RSA) women with ongoing pregnancies. They inferred that PCO and hyperandrogenism might be associated with recurring miscarriage. Hypersecretion of LH thus seems to be a critical issue in determining the reproductive outcome in women with PCO. The variable that is paramount in predicting pregnancy result is LH concentration in the conception cycle.

Mechanism

It is well known that normal and mildly elevated LH levels induce increased activity of ovarian 17-hydroxylase, 17,20-lyase, and the cytochrome P450c17a (P450) enzymes. It leads to increased ovarian 17a-hydroxyprogesterone (17-OHP) and androstenedione production. In contrast, it has been shown in both in vitro and in vivo studies in animals and in vitro studies in women that high LH concentrations have opposite effects on these enzymes. This LH downregulating effect appears to be more marked on 17,20-lyase than on 17-hydroxylase. Finally, these LH effects have not been reported in vivo in women. LH induces stimulating and downregulating effects on both ovarian D417-hydroxylase and D417,20-lyase activities as serum LH levels gradually increase. However, in contrast to in vitro studies, LH levels which induce P450 downregulation appears to be less effective on D417,20-lyase than on D417-hydroxylase in vivo. It strongly suggests that serum factors cause a marked increase in D417,20-lyase, but not in D417-hydroxylase, activity leading to both partial impairments of LH-induced D417,20-lyase downregulation and complete LH-induced D417-hydroxylase downregulation in these patients.[27] It is well known now that hypersecretion of LH leads to dysovulation, improper immunological attenuation of the implantation ambiance, and subsequent miscarriages.

Can Suppression of Luteinizing Hormone Improve Pregnancy Outcome?

Theoretically, suppression of LH should get better results in the treatment of infertility and pregnancy outcome. What needs to be evaluated is does this happen in reality. LH secretion can be suppressed by LH-releasing hormone (LHRH) analogs and antagonists. The use of LHRH analogs followed by HMG has been employed in IVF programs for tackling this problem of high LH.

Early reports did suggest that this may perk up the conception rates in women with PCO. In one study of women with anovulatory PCO-resistant to clomiphene citrate and high LH, the collective live-birth rate was considerably greater in those treated with LHRH analog and HMG when compared with those receiving HMG or FSH therapy unaccompanied.[28] It was achieved by a lower miscarriage rate in the LHRH analog group. However, other studies have not confirmed this advantage.[29,30] Thus, the use of LHRH analog in ovulation induction therapy is controversial.

Pituitary inhibition management has found a more scientific role in IVF regimes, with many studies reporting improved figures of oocytes obtained after superovulation, a lower incidence of premature luteinization, increased numbers of embryos transferred, improved pregnancy, and lower miscarriage rates.[31-33] Pituitary desensitization with LHRH analog therapy does have a useful effect on the outcome of pregnancies achieved after IVF, although this effect is less clear with ovulation induction therapy. There are no published data on the use of pituitary suppression of LH in ovulatory women who have PCO, hypersecretion of LH, and repeated miscarriage. Results of a small pilot study carried out suggest that LHRH agonist therapy followed by low-dose ovulation induction in women with recurrent miscarriage is an effective way of lowering LH and achieving a successful pregnancy.[34] Therefore, in clinical practice, it seems that suppression of LH may not be of much help, but it does help in IVF subjects.

POLYCYSTIC OVARIAN SYNDROME—INSULIN RESISTANCE AND RECURRENT PREGNANCY LOSS

It is undoubtedly the most intriguing and debated aspect of endocrinal causes of recurrent pregnancy failure. Heterogeneous and inconsistent interpretation of what is PCOS has further mired the situation. While high LH has been discussed at length in the previous section, it is insulin resistance that has also caught the attention of science in its role in the causation of recurrent miscarriages. In clinical practice, insulin resistance has been tackled with many good studies reporting favorable results. It is therefore understandable to visit this issue in this chapter. In a study of 197 subjects in whom the diagnosis of PCOS was confirmed on Rotterdam criteria (Table 6.1), these subjects were followed till the final outcome of pregnancy were achieved. Both groups were compared for risk of early pregnancy loss. It was found that continuation of metformin during pregnancy reduced early pregnancy loss, i.e. 8.8% versus 29.4% in cases and controls, respectively (p < 0.001). In the subset of women with a prior history of miscarriage, the pregnancy loss rate was 12.5% in the metformin versus 49.4% in control group.[35]

Table 6.1: Diagnostic criteria for PCOS.

NIH criteria (1990)	Rotterdam criteria (2003)	AES criteria (2006)
All three of the following: 1. Clinical or biochemical evidence of hyperandrogenism 2. Oligomenorrhea and/or anovulation 3. Exclusion of other disorders.	At least two of the following: 1. Oligomenorrhea and/or anovulation 2. Clinical and/or biochemical signs of hyperandrogenism 3. Polycystic ovaries.	All three of the following: 1. Hyperandrogenism (clinical or biochemical) 2. Ovarian dysfunction (oligomenorrhea or anovulation and/or polycystic ovarian morphology) 3. Exclusion of other androgen excess or related disorders.
	PCOS can be diagnosed only after the exclusion of related disorders (e.g. severe insulin resistance, androgen-secreting neoplasms and Cushing's syndrome, hyperprolactinemia, and thyroid abnormalities).	PCOS is predominantly a disorder of androgen excess.

(AES: Androgen Excess Society; NIH: National Institutes of Health; PCOS: Polycystic ovarian syndrome)

In an overview of the situation, one can say that despite the many studies that have investigated the prevalence of PCOS in recurrent miscarriage, the extent to which PCOS contributes remains highly uncertain. The majority of these studies have used the polycystic ovarian morphology alone to define PCOS, and the results are extremely variable due to a variety of diagnostic and selection criteria used. Only a tiny number of studies have investigated the prevalence of hyperandrogenemia in recurrent miscarriage. Most crucially, there is apparently not yet a single publication which has examined the actual prevalence of the complete syndrome of PCOS in recurrent miscarriage using the Rotterdam criteria. The possible mechanisms by which PCOS could cause recurrent miscarriage are considered: hyperandrogenemia, obesity, and hyperinsulinemia are the most likely candidates, although further work is needed. There is evidence to suggest that weight loss, ovarian drilling, and metformin up to about 14 weeks could help to reduce the rate of miscarriage.[36]

Case Study

Mrs RS had PCOS as per Rotterdam criteria. Her first three pregnancies ended in spontaneous miscarriages at 6 weeks, 8 weeks, and 6 weeks of pregnancy, respectively. All these were at other hospitals. After this, she came to us for care. Her next pregnancy was a conception following ovulation induction with clomiphene citrate. Metformin was continued from her prepregnancy phase when on a treatment of infertility till 14 weeks of pregnancy after which it was discontinued. That pregnancy went on uneventfully, and she had a full-term live delivery at 38 weeks normally.

In her subsequent pregnancy, she had a spontaneous conception. No ovulogens or metformin was used as it was a spontaneous conception. She presented to us with 6 weeks pregnant and bleeding per vagina. Her sonography picture is as shown in Figure 6.1. The fetal pole was not visible as yet.

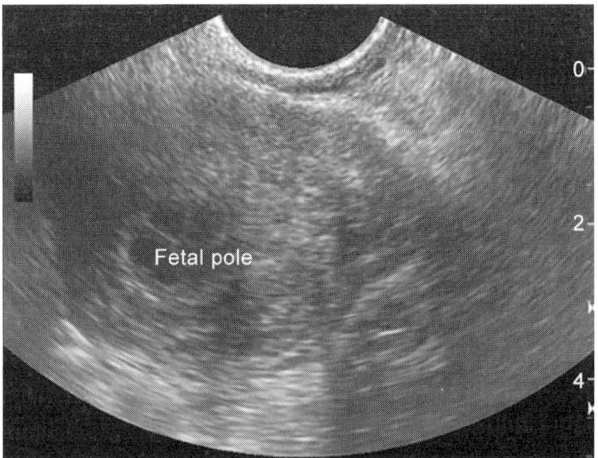

Fig. 6.1: 6 weeks pregnancy: Absent fetal pole.

There were areas of subchorionic hemorrhage as seen in Figure 6.2.

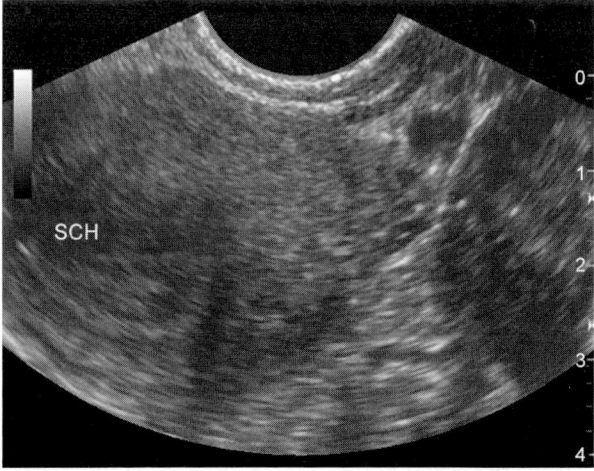

Fig. 6.2: 6 weeks pregnancy: Diffuse areas of subchorionic hemorrhage (SCH).

After 1 week, on follow-up, the gestational sac had increased in size but still fetal pole was not yet seen as shown in Figure 6.3. The prognosis was explained.

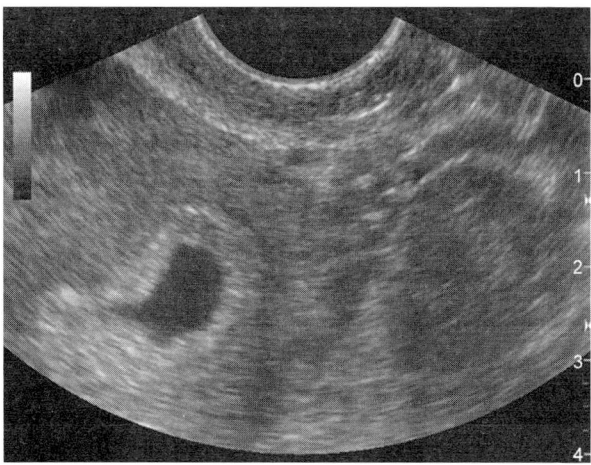

Fig. 6.3: At 7 weeks: Gestational sac increased in size but fetal pole still not seen.

After 1 week at the gestational age of 8 weeks of pregnancy fetal pole could be seen and fetal heart activity also became obvious. However, as shown in Figure 6.4 the heart rate was slow. She was explained the likely outcome and was told that this conception may be lost.

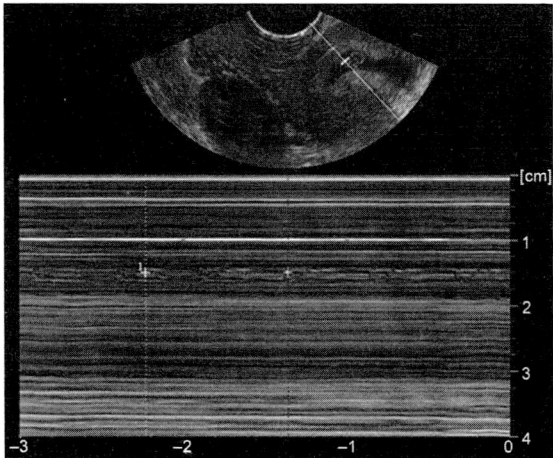

Fig. 6.4: At 8 weeks: Slow heart rate.

At 10 weeks she had absent fetal heart activity as seen in Figure 6.5 though the fetal configuration was well seen.

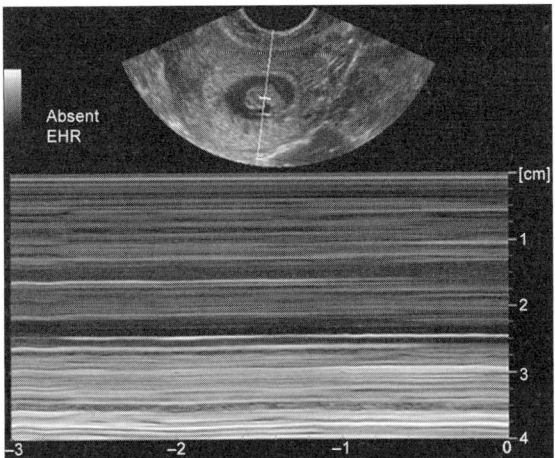

Fig. 6.5: At 9 weeks: Absent heart activity.

Polycystic ovary is clearly visible in Figure 6.6.

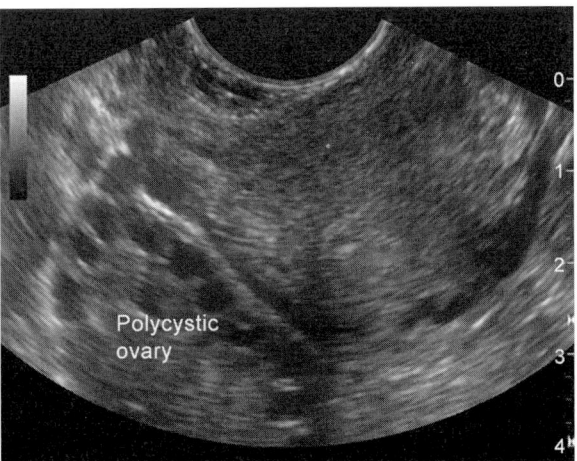

Fig. 6.6: Polycystic ovary.

On subsequent follow-up, she was proved to have insulin resistance on investigations. She was treated with metformin in a dose of 650 milligrams twice a day. She had a spontaneous conception. Metformin was continued for 14 weeks of pregnancy. She went on to deliver normally a full-term live child of optimum weight.

SUGGESTED READING

- Recurrent Miscarriages by Desai P, Patel P; Academia Publishers: Delhi from which this chapter draws on many points and is duly acknowledged.

REFERENCES

1. Arredondo F, Noble LS. Endocrinology of recurrent pregnancy loss. Semin Reprod Med. 2006;24(1):33-9.
2. Mills JL, Simpson JL, Driscoll SG, et al. Incidence of spontaneous abortion among normal women and insulin-dependent diabetic women whose pregnancies were identified within 21 days of conception. N Engl J Med. 1988;319(25):1617-23.
3. Hanson U, Perrson B, Thunnel S. Relationship between Hb1ac in diabetic pregnancy and obstetric outcome. Diabetologia. 1990;33:100-4.
4. Miodovnik M, Skillman C, Holroyde JC, et al. Elevated maternal glycohemoglobin in early pregnancy and spontaneous abortion among insulin-dependent diabetic women. Am J Obstet Gynecol. 1985;153(4):439-42.
5. Miodovnik M, Mimouni F, Siddiqi TA, et al. Spontaneous abortions in repeat diabetic pregnancies: a relationship with glycemic control. Obstet Gynecol. 1990;75(1):75-8.
6. Stray-Pedersen B, Stray-Pedersen S. Etiologic factors and subsequent reproductive performance in 195 couples with a prior history of habitual abortion. Am J Obstet Gynecol. 1984;148(2):140-6.
7. Winikoff D, Malinek M. The predictive value of thyroid "test profile" in habitual abortion. Br J Obstet Gynaecol. 1975;82(9):760-6.
8. Clifford K, Rai R, Watson H, et al. An informative protocol for the investigation of recurrent miscarriage: preliminary experience of 500 consecutive cases. Hum Reprod. 1994;9(7):1328-32.
9. Poorolajal J, Cheraghi P, Cheraghi Z, et al. Predictors of miscarriage: a matched case-control study. Epidemiol Health. 2014;36:e2014031.

10. Bernardi LA, Cohen RN, Stephenson MD. Impact of subclinical hypothyroidism in women with recurrent early pregnancy loss. Fertil Steril. 2013;100(5):1326-31.
11. Di Renzo GC, Giardina I, Clerici G, et al. Progesterone in normal and pathological pregnancy. Horm Mol Biol Clin Investig. 2016;27(1):35-48.
12. Wang SW, Ma LL, Huang S, et al. Role of Cervical Cerclage and Vaginal Progesterone in the Treatment of Cervical Incompetence with/without Preterm Birth History. Chin Med J (Engl). 2016;129(22):2670-5.
13. Corner GW, Allen WM. Physiology of the corpus luteum. 1929. Am J Obstet Gynecol. 2005;193(4):1574.
14. Serle E, Aplin JD, Li TC, et al. Endometrial differentiation in the peri-implantation phase of women with recurrent miscarriage: a morphological and immunohistochemical study. Fertil Steril. 1994;62(5):989-96.
15. Csapo AI Pulkinnen MO, Wiest WG. Effects of luteectomy and progesterone replacement therapy in early pregnant patients. Am J Obstet Gynecol. 1973;115(6):759-65.
16. Vignali M, Centinaio G. Efficacy of the vaginal administration of natural progesterone in patients with recurrent spontaneous hormone caused abortion. Minerva Ginecol. 2000;52(9):367-74.
17. Fritz MA. Inadequate luteal function and recurrent abortion. Semin Reprod Endocrinol. 1988;6:129-43.
18. Li TC, Cooke ID. Review: Evaluation of the luteal phase. Hum Reprod. 1991;6(4):484-99.
19. Daya S, Gunby J. Luteal phase support in assisted reproduction cycles. Cochrane Database Syst Rev. 2004;(3):CD004830.
20. Desai P. Prevention of preeclampsia and other obstetric vasculopathies. In: Desai P (Ed). Obstetric Vasculopathies, 1st edition. New Delhi: Jaypee Brothers Medical Publishers (P) Ltd; 2013. p. 75.
21. Morley LC, Simpson N, Tang T. Human chorionic gonadotrophin (hCG) for preventing miscarriage. Cochrane Database Syst Rev. 2013;(1):CD008611.
22. Daya S. Efficacy of progesterone support for pregnancy in women with recurrent miscarriage. A meta-analysis of controlled trials. Br J Obstet Gynaecol. 1989;96(3):275-80.
23. Haas DM, Ramsey PS. Progestogen for preventing miscarriage. Cochrane Database Syst Rev. 2013;(10):CD003511.
24. El-Zibdeh MY. Dydrogesterone in the reduction of recurrent spontaneous abortion. J Steroid Biochem Mol Biol. 2005;97(5):431-4.
25. Carp H. A systematic review of dydrogesterone for the treatment of recurrent miscarriage. Gynecol Endocrinol. 2015;31(6):422-30.

26. Tulppala M, Stenman UH, Cacciatore B, et al. Polycystic ovaries and levels of gonadotrophins and androgens in recurrent miscarriage: prospective study in 50 women. Br J Obstet Gynaecol. 1993;100(4):348-52.
27. Leigh AJ, Peattie AB. Polycystic ovaries and levels of gonadotrophins and androgens in recurrent miscarriage: prospective study in 50 women. Br J Obstet Gynecol. 1994;101(3):275-6.
28. Farhi J, Homburg R, Lerner A, et al. The choice of treatment for anovulation associated with polycystic ovary syndrome following failure to conceive with clomiphene. Hum Reprod. 1993;8(9):1367-71.
29. Charbonnel B, Krempf M, Blanchard P, et al. Induction of ovulation in polycystic ovary syndrome with a combination of a luteinizing hormone-releasing hormone analog and exogenous gonadotropins. Fertil Steril. 1987;47(6):920-4.
30. Homburg R, Eshel A, Kilborn J, et al. Combined luteinizing hormone releasing hormone analogue and exogenous gonadotrophins for the treatment of infertility associated with polycystic ovaries. Hum Reprod. 1990;5(1):32-5.
31. Antoine JM, Salat-Baroux J, Alvarez S, et al. Ovarian stimulation using human menopausal gonadotrophins with or without LHRH analogues in a long protocol for in-vitro fertilization: a prospective randomized comparison. Hum Reprod. 1990;5(5):565-9.
32. Frydman R, Fries N, Belaisch-Allart JC, et al. Luteinizing hormone-releasing hormone agonists in in vitro fertilization: Different methods of utilization and comparison with previous ovulation stimulation treatments. Hum Reprod. 1988;3:559-61.
33. Rutherford AJ, Subak-Sharpe RJ, Dawson KJ, et al. Improvement in vitro fertilisation after treatment with buserelin, an agonist of luteinising hormone releasing hormone. Br Med J (Clin Res Ed). 1988;296(6639):1765-8.
34. Watson H, Kiddy DS, Hamilton-Fairley D, et al. Hypersecretion of luteinizing hormone and ovarian steroids in women with recurrent early miscarriage. Hum Reprod. 1993;8(6):829-33.
35. Nawaz FH, Rizvi J. Continuation of metformin reduces early pregnancy loss in obese Pakistani women with polycystic ovarian syndrome. Gynecol Obstet Invest. 2010;69(3):184-9.
36. Cocksedge KA, Li TC, Saravelos SH, et al. A reappraisal of the role of polycystic ovary syndrome in recurrent miscarriage. Reprod Biomed Online. 2008;17(1):151-60.

Chapter 7

Endometriosis and Recurrent Spontaneous Miscarriages

INTRODUCTION

The association between endometriosis and spontaneous miscarriages remains hazy and vague. This chapter reviews the controversies around this area in the light of new literature. As early as in 1942 there was a hint of an association between endometriosis and recurrent spontaneous miscarriages.[1] Expectedly this started many reviews and studies to establish the connection, if any, between the two conditions. About 3 decades ago endometriosis was listed among the established causes of spontaneous miscarriages.[2,3] However, since then, convincing evidence of the association between the two is still not forthcoming.

ENDOMETRIOSIS AND PREGNANCY LOSS—EXAMINING THE EVIDENCE

When one attempts to examine evidence, one striking feature that catches the eye is that many of these studies are retrospective. In one of these studies, the incidence of endometriosis is determined by prelaparoscopy incidence of spontaneous miscarriage, patients treated for endometriosis by laparoscopic surgery, and then the posttreatment incidence of spontaneous miscarriage during postsurgical follow-up was determined.[4] This study found that there seems to be an association of 1st trimester spontaneous miscarriage and untreated endometriosis. In this report, 52% of an untreated group of patients with endometriosis aborted. However, 12% of the second group of surgically treated patients and 7% of the third group of patients treated with danazol aborted. Therefore, medical or surgical therapy for endometriosis lowered the miscarriage rate significantly. Within 2 years of publication of this study, another study got published in which the average spontaneous miscarriage rate before the diagnosis of endometriosis for all patients was 63.1%. After surgical treatment, the miscarriage rate dropped to 0% ($p < 0.000001$) for all stages of the disease. However, even in those patients who received expectant management only, the miscarriage rate fell from the group average 63.1% to 16.7% and 21.4% for mild and moderate endometriosis, respectively ($p < 0.001$).[5] These results suggest that the spontaneous miscarriage rate in untreated endometriosis may not be as high as previously reported and may not be significantly different from the rate in the general population.[5] Miscarriage rates dropping to 0% posttreatment should be viewed very carefully and with necessary vigilance. Interestingly no other study has produced such astounding results after that.

In another study by Chinese workers, it has been suggested that it is considered that the infertility of patients with minimal to mild endometriosis is associated with the alteration of the pelvic microenvironment. Several kinds of cytokines and proteins are involved in this process.[6] They may disturb steps necessary to achieve a successful pregnancy, such as ovulation, gamete transport, fertilization, embryo transport, and implantation. Extrapolating, these authors have suggested that any disturbance to one of the steps mentioned earlier may lead to pregnancy loss.[6]

In a recent cohort study from Canada spread over 12 years, some interesting results have been published. The aim of this study was to provide a temporal-spatial reference of adverse pregnancy outcomes (APOs) and examine whether endometriosis promotes APO in the same population. Among the 31,068 women who had a pregnancy between 1997 and 2008 in Eastern Townships of Canada, 6,749 (21.7%) had APO. Among the 31,068 pregnancies, 784 (2.5%) had endometriosis, and 183 (23.3%) had both endometriosis and APO. Endometriosis has been shown to increase the incidence of fetal loss including spontaneous miscarriage and stillbirth.[7]

POSSIBLE CAUSES OF ENDOMETRIOSIS AND PREGNANCY LOSS

The quality of evidence for an association between endometriosis and recurrent pregnancy loss is at best vague. As a result trying to explain why endometriosis (if at all) causes pregnancy loss is a difficult exercise. As regards the microenvironment mentioned in previous paragraphs, an interesting study has emerged recently. Micro ribonucleic acid (miRNA) has emerged as important epigenetic modulators of gene expression in diverse pathological and physiological processes. In the endometrium, miRNA appears to have a role in the dynamic changes associated with the menstrual cycle, in implantation, and the pathophysiology associated with reproductive disorders such as recurrent miscarriage and endometriosis. This review explores the role of miRNA in endometrial physiology and endometrial disorders of reproduction and also raises the prospect that circulating miRNA may modulate endometrial function or reflect disordered endometrial activity. miRNA is small RNA fragments that suppress the production of specific proteins to alter cell behavior in a particular way. miRNA is also able to travel in the blood and change the function of distant cells. miRNA has been identified in endometrial tissues and blood and appears to participate in the cellular alterations associated with implantation, recurrent miscarriage, and endometriosis.[8]

Immunology may also be holding some clue here. In this, macrophages seem to have some role. Macrophage function has been under a close study in endometriosis for long. One recent study has tried to examine its role in recurrent miscarriages. Macrophages hold a pivotal role in both regulating and executing the body's immune response under various conditions. Hence, although endometriosis, preeclampsia, and miscarriages are clinically different, all three are regarded to involve highly complex immunological processes. In this study, macrophages have been shown to invade endometriosis lesions and to mediate propagation of endometriotic cyst growth. Also, a significant G protein-coupled estrogen receptor (GPER) upregulation in macrophages is demonstrated in this study. It highlights a potential alternative way through which estrogen may modulate the immune response of macrophages in endometriosis. Also, during spontaneous miscarriages, the macrophage population increases significantly. This deregulation may support an inflammatory scheme further triggering the abortive process.[9]

Natural killer cells also known as NK cells have an important role in the immunology of pregnancy. They have also been thought to play a vital role in endometriosis. Women, with or without endometriosis, who have larger populations of cytotoxic CD16(+) NK cells or higher populations of NKp46(+), CD56(+) cells may be at greater risk of infertility disorders resulting from an inflammatory environment occurring during implantation or later during decidualization.[10] However, to what extent do they play a role in recurrent miscarriage is still unknown.

There is apparently an endocrine association to endometriosis and miscarriages. It is a well-known fact that there is some association between endometriosis and luteal phase defect. Luteal phase defect is a result of alteration in corpus luteum function. The well-known essential functions of corpus luteum are nidation and support of early pregnancy. Any defect in its function can lead to loss of pregnancies.

Another interesting postulate associating endometriosis with pregnancy failures was related to the quality of the oocyte in endometriosis. Several studies have shown that the quality of oocytes retrieved in subjects with endometriosis is suboptimal.[11-13] However, extrapolating this to an increased possibility of miscarriages in endometriosis may not necessarily be true. In one of the recent articles, a review of how endometriosis affects the development of each stage of reproductive life from conception to birth has been done. At the end, the authors conclude that more research is needed to study the biological pathways of the fertility impairment caused by this disease.[14]

To sum up therefore, there appears to be a strong case for endometriosis to be associated with pregnancy loss recurrent or otherwise. The basis of this could be immunological and endocrinal or both. However, when evidence is carefully examined, it appears that there is no increase in rates of miscarriages in subjects with endometriosis. Nevertheless, it must also be accepted that endometriosis still has many hidden facets. It is, therefore, possible that over a period of time these aspects may get revealed and conclusions may change. But as of now, it is safe to conclude that there is hardly any association between endometriosis and recurrent or anecdotal spontaneous pregnancy loss.

ENDNOTE

While revising this chapter for this new edition, there was a dilemma as to whether it should be retained at all. It is because in the time that has elapsed between the previous edition and this one the blurry picture has hardly cleared anymore. The reason it has been retained is to review the controversies around this area of association between endometriosis and miscarriages in the light of new literature.

REFERENCES

1. Haydon GB. A study of 569 cases of endometriosis. Am J Obstet Gynecol. 1942;43(4):704-9.
2. Naples JD, Batt RE, Sadigh H. Spontaneous abortion rate in patients with endometriosis. Obstet Gynecol. 1981;57:509-12.
3. Wheeler JM, Johnston BM, Malinak LR. The relationship of endometriosis to spontaneous abortion. Fertil Steril. 1983;39(5):656-60.
4. Groll M. Endometriosis and spontaneous abortion. Fertil Steril. 1984;41(6):933-5.
5. Metzger DA, Olive DL, Stohs GF, et al. Association of endometriosis and spontaneous abortion: effect of control group selection. Fertil Steril. 1986;45(1):18-22.
6. Chen XJ, Huang HF. Research on minimal to mild endometriosis associated infertility. Zhejiang Da Xue Xue Bao Yi Xue Ban. 2007;36(5):515-20.
7. Aris A. A 12-year cohort study on adverse pregnancy outcomes in Eastern Townships of Canada: impact of endometriosis. Gynecol Endocrinol. 2014;30(1):34-7.
8. Hull ML, Nisenblat V. Tissue and circulating microRNA influence reproductive function in endometrial disease. Reprod Biomed Online. 2013;27(5):515-29.

9. Hutter S, Heublein S, Knabl J, et al. Macrophages: are they involved in endometriosis, abortion and preeclampsia and how? J Nippon Med Sch. 2013;80(2):97-103.
10. Giuliani E, Parkin KL, Lessey BA, et al. Characterization of uterine NK cells in women with infertility or recurrent pregnancy loss and associated endometriosis. Am J Reprod Immunol. 2014;72(3):262-9.
11. Da Broi MG, Malvezzi H, Paz CC, et al. Follicular fluid from infertile women with mild endometriosis may compromise the meiotic spindles of bovine metaphase II oocytes. Hum Reprod. 2014;29(2):315-23.
12. Dong X, Liao X, Wang R, et al. The impact of endometriosis on IVF/ICSI outcomes. Int J Clin Exp Pathol. 2013;6(9):1911-8.
13. Hauzman EE, Garcia-Velasco JA, Pellicer A. Oocyte donation and endometriosis: What are the lessons? Semin Reprod Med. 2013;31(2):173-7.
14. Carvalho LF, Rossener R, Azeem A, et al. From conception to birth—how endometriosis affects the development of each stage of reproductive life. Minerva Ginecol. 2013;65(2):181-98.

Chapter 8

Infections and Recurrent Spontaneous Miscarriages

INTRODUCTION

Among so many infections that have been blamed for recurrent pregnancy miscarriages, TORCH infections have been the most consistent. TORCH stands for T—Toxoplasmosis, O—Other infections, R—Rubella, C—Cytomegalovirus, and H—Herpes simplex virus-2. The "other agents" under O include coxsackievirus, chickenpox (caused by varicella zoster virus), parvovirus B19, chlamydia, human immunodeficiency virus (HIV), human T-lymphotropic virus, and syphilis. For quite sometime TORCH enjoyed the popularity as one of the most commonly investigated etiological factor of recurrent miscarriages. But expectedly scientific investigations supervened to disprove any role of these infections in causing recurrent miscarriages. It has now gone off the request list of any good obstetrician. Two studies both by the same lead author find some role for investigating subjects with recurrent miscarriages.[1,2] Both studies suffer from a significant handicap of petite sample size. So as of now the current thinking that TORCH does not produce recurrent miscarriages holds true. The author has since last 2 decades or more not subjected any woman with a recurrent spontaneous miscarriage to TORCH testing, and we find no need to change this policy.

Besides TORCH, a number of organisms have been implicated at one time or the other as etiological for recurrent pregnancy loss (RPL). They have been summarized in Table 8.1.

Table 8.1: Organisms associated (but not proved) with spontaneous miscarriages.

Viruses	Bacteria	Spirochetes	Parasites
Cytomegalovirus	Listeria monocytogenes	Treponema pallidum	Toxoplasma gondii
Rubella	Ureaplasma urealyticum		Plasmodium falciparum
Herpes simplex	Mycoplasma hominis		
Human immuno-deficiency virus	Bacterial vaginosis		
	Chlamydia trachomatis		

How do Infections Cause Recurrent Pregnancy Loss (RPL) if at All?

It was postulated that these organisms or their products directly or indirectly provoke the conversion of arachidonic acid in the decidua into prostaglandins (PGE2 and PGF2α). These prostaglandins produce uterine contractions and subsequent miscarriage. Another mechanism postulated was mediated through cytokines. One recent study has indicated that polarization of macrophages and modulation of Th subsets could contribute to trophoblast apoptosis through different mechanisms thereby leading to miscarriage.[3]

It has been well known that premature rupture of membranes (PROMs) has an association with chorioamnionitis and cytokines. Nevertheless, whether this is a cause-effect relationship or is a result of the same cause is far from clear. But this association between cytokines, rupture of membranes, and chorioamnionitis led to a postulate that this was also the cause of recurrent spontaneous miscarriages. One such study tried to determine whether amniotic fluid (AF) inflammation, in the absence of infection, is associated with adverse pregnancy outcomes in nonelective cervical cerclage patients.[4] They found that elevated AF white blood cell (WBC) count was correlated with severe and extreme preterm delivery. Decreased AF glucose was associated with histological chorioamnionitis and a decreased cerclage to the birth interval. Elevated AF interleukin-6

(IL-6) correlated significantly with decreased gestational age at delivery and reduced cerclage to the delivery interval in this study. High IL-6 concentrations were associated with severe, extreme preterm delivery, and neonatal death. This study, however, could not prove the association of infections with recurring adverse pregnancy outcomes. It is therefore understandable that a series of workers doubt the role of infections in recurrent spontaneous miscarriages.[5-8]

The consequence of infection on pregnancy outcome depends on some factors, such as the quantity and virulence of the organism implicated, the place of the inoculum, the duration of gestation, the resulting fetal and placental injury, and the mother's resistance response. Any infection that can cause morbidities like fever may bring on a miscarriage. In repeated miscarriages, the organisms assumed to be causing repeated fetal loss that have to prevail subclinically in the mother for a long time to evade a diagnosis and treatment. But there is no persuasive proof that any of the infections that have been implicated at some point or the other can cause recurrent spontaneous miscarriages.

It has become necessary to review one study recently published which tries to prove that chronic endometritis due to common bacteria is prevalent in women with recurrent miscarriage as confirmed by improved pregnancy outcome after antibiotic treatment.[9] This study is only one of its kind. No other studies have shown such fabulous results with antibiotics use. The subgroups are handicapped by small numbers. The authors seem to have started with a bias, and there are many design flaws in the study. As of now this study has to be archived till that time as new and numerous studies get published corroborating these findings but with better study design.[10]

ESSENTIALS OF LABORATORY DIAGNOSIS FOR PROVING THE ASSOCIATION BETWEEN SPECIFIC ORGANISM AND RECURRENT PREGNANCY LOSS

The diagnosis relies on recognition of the organisms in the products or placental bed to connect a particular microbe to miscarriage.

Till date, culture seems to be the most reliable technique. But now, antigen detection and polymerase chain reaction (PCR) are emerging methods. Detection of the same organism in consecutive miscarriages is the testimony to that infectious organism. A different method for linking an infectious agent with the condition can be the demonstration of the expression of specific antibodies when the miscarriage is happening. A high antibody titer, nevertheless, shows that an infection has occurred at some instance of time. It does not, however, say when the infection may have occurred. To prove a contributory association between an infectious agent and RPL by serologic means is therefore difficult. So, routine antibody study of patients with a history of recurrent spontaneous miscarriages is not justified. In fact, most couples with recurrent miscarriage do not benefit from an extensive diagnostic workup for infections. Also clinicians at times do not understand how to interpret these results adding further to the problem. Their response after that is to treat empirically, which is neither justified nor rational.

SPECIFIC INFECTIONS AND RECURRENT PREGNANCY LOSS

We shall now examine the role of specific infections in causing recurrent spontaneous miscarriages if at all.

Chlamydia Trachomatis

These organisms are known to infect human reproductive tract. 2–20% of asymptomatic mothers have been estimated to be affected by *Chlamydia trachomatis*. Though its role in infertility and ectopic pregnancy is well examined, its role in recurrent spontaneous miscarriages remains dubious.[7-10] One important study has proved the association between *Chlamydia trachomatis* infection and sensory-neural hearing loss in newborn.[11] However, its role as a cause of recurrent spontaneous miscarriages is not established.

Bacterial Vaginosis

Interest in bacterial vaginosis (BV) arose from its association with preterm birth. One study has hinted at an increased risk of pregnancy loss and BV.[12] But it too did not find an immediate association between recurrent spontaneous miscarriages and BV. In fact, there are hardly any studies that examine the association between RPL and BV. This author does not carry out screening for BV in his subjects with RPL.

Genital Mycoplasma

A study that reportedly isolated *Mycoplasma hominis* and *Ureaplasma urealyticum* from the vagina of 40-70% of pregnant woman paved the way for postulating an association between fungal infections and RPL.[13] Support for this came from studies as early as in 1970.[6-11] These studies found some association between *Ureaplasma* infection and sporadic miscarriages (but not recurrent spontaneous miscarriages). One study found evidence of *Ureaplasma urealyticum* in endometrial biopsies of subjects with recurrent losses.[14] These biopsies were not taken when they were aborting but after the episode. This weak point degraded the quality of evidence. Studies that show beneficial results in subjects treated with anti-infective agents are not much of help as they are not randomized controlled trials. Hence as of now, there is no reason to recommend either a routine screen or empirical treatment for these conditions in subjects with RPL.

Coxiella Burnetii

This organism causes the common zoonotic disease Q fever. It is commonly found in areas where breeding of livestock is undertaken. One study from Turkey hinted that *Coxiella burnetii* could cause miscarriage during the 1st trimester, while at later stages it tends to become chronic causing low-birth weight babies and premature birth.[15] This study further went on to suggest that in regions where livestock breeding is common in cases with recurrent miscarriage and premature births, women and their husbands should be screened for *Coxiella burnetii*. Apparently, these authors have used sound scientific methods of study, but they seem to have started with a bias. This bias being that *Coxiella burnetii* causes specified adverse obstetric outcomes.

Another larger and more systematic study from Denmark nevertheless completely dispels this conclusion. The authors of this study claim that theirs is the first population-based seroepidemiologic study evaluating pregnancy outcome in women with serologically verified exposure to *Coxiella burnetii* against a comparable reference group of seronegative women. These authors found no increased risk of adverse pregnancy outcome in women with confirmed exposure to *Coxiella burnetii*.[16]

Waddlia Chondrophila

Baud D et al. investigated the zoonotic potential of Waddlia chondrophila which is a new chlamydia-like organism as an abortigenic agent.[17] Though the seroprevalence was higher in women with sporadic and recurrent miscarriages, whether this can be translated into clinical practice, needs to be studied. Therefore as of now, our perception that RPL is not associated with any infecting agent still holds true.

Are Antiphospholipid Antibodies Originating in Infections?

The need for this question arose by following some recent studies that suggest that infections can include antiphospholipid (APL) antibodies. Besides infection, genetics and trauma have also been implicated in the induction of APL. They have postulated that in a genetically susceptible individual, exposure to one or more infectious agent can cause a molecular mimicry and result in the production of pathogenic APL and their subsequent effects.[18] However, it is still too early to either support or refute this association between APL and RPL.

REFERENCES

1. Kishore J, Gupta I. Serological study of parvovirus B19 infection in women with recurrent spontaneous abortions. Indian J Pathol Microbiol. 2006;49(4):548-50.
2. Kishore J, Agarwal J, Agrawal S, et al. Seroanalysis of Chlamydia trachomatis and S-TORCH agents in women with recurrent spontaneous abortions. Indian J Pathol Microbiol. 2003;46(4):684-7.

3. Liu T, Zhang Q, Liu L, et al. Trophoblast apoptosis through polarization of macrophages induced by Chinese Toxoplasma gondii isolates with different virulence in pregnant mice. Parasitol Res. 2013;112(8):3019-27.
4. Aguin F, Aguin T, Cordoba M, et al. Amniotic fluid inflammation with negative culture and outcome after cervical cerclage. J Matern Fetal Neonatal Med. 2012;25(10):1990-4.
5. Capal E, Salomon F, Somploinski D. Early miscarriage and mycoplasma infection. Isr J Med Sci. 1972;8(2):122-7.
6. Gray DJ, Robinson HB, Malone J, et al. Adverse outcome in pregnancy following amniotic fluid isolation of Ureaplasma urealyticum. Prenatal Diagn. 1992;12(2):111-7.
7. Grönroos M, Honkonen E, Terho P, et al. Cervical and serum IgA and serum IgG antibodies to Chlamydia trachomatis and herpes simplex virus in threatening abortion: a prospective study. Br J Obstet Gynaecol. 1983;90(2):167-70.
8. Gump DW, Gibson M, Ashikaga T. Lack of association between mycoplasmas and infertility. N Engl J Med. 1984;310(15):937-41.
9. Cicinelli E, Matteo M, Tinelli R, et al. Chronic endometritis due to common bacteria is prevalent in women with recurrent miscarriage as confirmed by improved pregnancy outcome after antibiotic treatment. Reprod Sci. 2014;21(5):640-7.
10. Munday PE, Porter R, Falder PF, et al. Spontaneous abortion—an infectious aetiology? Br J Obstet Gynaecol. 1984;91(12):1177-80.
11. Mosca F, Pugni L. Cytomegalovirus infection: the state of the art. J Chemother. 2007;19 Suppl 2:46-8.
12. McGregor JA, French JI, Parker R, et al. Prevention of premature birth by screening and treatment of common genital tract infections: results of a prospective controlled evaluation. Am J Obstet Gynecol. 1995;173(1):157-67.
13. Witkin SS, Sultan KM, Neal GS, et al. Unsuspected Chlamydia trachomatis infection and in vitro fertilization outcome. Am J Obstet Gynecol. 1994;171(5):1208-14.
14. Stray-Pedersen B, Eng J, Reikvam TM. Uterine T-mycoplasma colonization in reproductive failure. Am J Obstet Gynecol. 1978;130(3):307-11.
15. Eyigör M, Gültekin B, Telli M, et al. Investigation of Coxiella burnetii prevalence in women who had miscarriage and their spouses by serological and molecular methods. Mikrobiyol Bul. 2013;47(2):324-31.
16. Nielsen SY, Andersen AM., Mølbak K, et al. No excess risk of adverse pregnancy outcomes among women with serological markers of

previous infection with *Coxiella burnetii*: evidence from the Danish National Birth Cohort. BMC Infect Dis. 2013;13:87.
17. Baud D, Thomas V, Arafa A, et al. Waddlia chondrophila, a potential agent of human fetal death. Emerg Infect Dis. 2007;13(8):1239-43.
18. Sherer Y, Blank M, Shoenfeld Y. Antiphospholipid syndrome (APS): where does it come from? Best Pract Res Clin Rheumatol. 2007;21(6):1071-8.

Chapter 9

Psychological Bearings of Recurrent Miscarriages

INTRODUCTION

Available current literature indicates that recurrent miscarriages can produce profound psychological effects on the subject. Respondents to one survey believed that miscarriage is a rare complication of pregnancy, with the majority believing that it occurred in 5% or less of all pregnancies.[1] There were also widespread misconceptions about causes of miscarriage. Those who had experienced a miscarriage often felt guilty, isolated, and alone. Identifying a potential cause of the miscarriage may affect patient's psychological and emotional responses.[1] Psychological responses seem to be the effect rather than the cause of recurrent miscarriage. As a result, providing systematic psychological support helps in getting better results with other treatment modalities in subjects with recurrent miscarriages. Recurrent spontaneous miscarriage has profound psychological effects even on the male partner. Psychological functioning, sexual satisfaction, and erectile function are impaired in these men.[2]

Most studies into psychological bearings of recurrent spontaneous miscarriages paid attention to the personality characteristics of the patients only and excluded other psychological factors.[3-8] Further, images of the personality characteristics of these patients are inclined to be stuck in the psychoanalytic hypothesis, which was popular at that time.

The literature describes women with miscarriage as high strung and tense emotionally volatile, uneasy, scared, and lacking in confidence and tear jerkers.[3] However, this seems to be a sweeping generalization and individualization is warranted. In a recent study, it ought to be underlined that not all women respond to miscarriage similarly. Women show a vast multiplicity of responses, and even though the bulk of women are saddened early after a miscarriage, they do not want or need grief psychotherapy as long as more conventional methods of support are employed. Factors predictive of an abnormal grief reaction include parity, bad marital association, prior pregnancy loss, prior psychiatric troubles, and the like. Unexpectedly, gestational age is not a factor.

IMMUNOLOGY, PSYCHOLOGY AND RECURRENT PREGNANCY LOSS

A possible connection between immunology and psychology are relatively new areas which are getting associated with recurrent pregnancy loss (RPL). It is a well-known fact that conditions like eczema and bronchial asthma are somatic manifestations of psychological causes and vice versa. Interestingly, some recent articles have tried to correlate the impact of psychology on natural killer (NK) cell activity and its bearing on recurrent spontaneous miscarriage. An Iranian group recognized that both acute and chronic conditions have a significant effect on the immune system. In conditions like depression, the immune system gets effectively downregulated.[9] They have also taken a cognizance of an association between depression and a higher number of circulating white blood cells (WBCs). They found a distinct association between a high-stress scare and NK cell activity. On the basis of their results they suggest that in subjects with recurrent spontaneous miscarriage, managing psychological aspects (stress/depression) can effectively alter the obstetric outcome in subjects with RPL.

With estimated 8.6% depression prevalence among subjects with recurrent spontaneous miscarriage,[10] one study found a different correlation between neurotic behavior and NK cell activity. It concluded that in addition to several substances such as transforming growth factor and granulocyte-macrophage colony-stimulating factor, depression scale score, and high self esteem contributed to high NK activity in women with recurrent spontaneous miscarriage.[11]

Further to this association between recurrent miscarriages, immunology, and psychological bearings it has been found that acute stress may have a stimulating effect on the immune system, while in the case of chronic stress especially depression, the immune system could be downregulated. However, an association between depression and a higher number of circulating WBCs with increased activity has been reported. Elevation in immune cell numbers and alteration in cytokine profiles are documented for women suffering from sporadic spontaneous miscarriage with a high-stress score.[9] This study goes on to suggest that psychological support will successfully modify the outcome in subjects with recurrent miscarriages. Similar immunological bearings in subjects of recurrent miscarriages were also shown in one earlier study.[12]

PROVIDING PSYCHOLOGICAL SUPPORT TO SUBJECTS WITH RECURRENT PREGNANCY LOSS

The concept of "human touch" is as relevant in subjects with recurrent spontaneous miscarriages as in other conditions of medicine. With widespread interconnectivity now suggested between immunology and psychological bearings in subjects with recurrent miscarriages, this support becomes all the more pertinent. It was from here that the concept of tender loving care (TLC) came into light.

Tender loving care consists of:
- Psychological support and weekly medical and ultrasonography (USG) examination.
- After a loss, provide feedback about potential reasons for the loss and information about the future.
- Reassurance to reduce apprehension.
- A follow-up visit after 2 weeks to share medical information and counseling about normal responses in the form of sadness, guilt and anger, depression, lack of concentration, and difficulty at work.
- In a case of significant depression beyond 4–6 months referral to an informed professional counselor and others with similar losses. Statistics indicate that even after a pregnancy loss the

chances for a live-born child with the next pregnancy are significantly high. Guidelines on the psychological management of recurrent spontaneous miscarriage have advised to give information on the pain process, tell subjects of the necessity to mourn, give past ultrasound pictures of what the fetus may have appeared like, and serve a psychotherapy function.[8,13-16] These guidelines may be apt for some women; a universal approach is necessary for the emotional support of patients with recurrent spontaneous miscarriages. The following three guiding principles are suggested:

1. Start recognizing of the psychological aspects of recurrent spontaneous miscarriage.
2. Provide detailed medical information.
3. Offer her reference to the mental health professional.

COMPONENTS OF SUPPORT GIVING THAT MAY BE HELPFUL

Same Caregivers

Seemingly very trivial matter, it has been found that for the success of this system, the same set of caregivers is essential. The team should make every attempt to serve as a constant team.

Frequent Visits

The rationale of this is to ask how she is responding and perceiving, whether or not she is worried, and whether she has any features. At the same time, frequent visits generate a feeling of being taken care of and provide an opportunity to answer any queries and reassure her.

Ample Patient Education

The caring doctor must make every effort to teach the patient about the medical cause and management of her particular problem in the interval period. All confusions should be enquired for and weeded out. A clear perception of what has gone wrong helps to lessen apprehensions. Reduction of these fears and generating a high level of confidence in the patient for her successful reproductive capacity should be the critical goal of this therapy.

When to Refer to a Psychotherapist?

If the subject has profound and far-reaching emotional effects, a reference will provide an atmosphere for dealing with these effects. Also, these subjects may also be having infertility, which can have a profound effect on sexuality, marriage, and family function. It can be lowering her self belief and self respect. Psychotherapy generates a setting for recognizing and identifying these in depth. Pregnancy itself is an unsure, emotional phase for lots of women. It is made particularly so with repetitive miscarriages. The right sort of psychotherapy can help the subjects to handle these aspects better and more scientifically.

TO SUM-UP

All in all what Javert said as early as in 1949 is still true, the perhaps nowhere in the fields of medicine does one encounter as many emotionally unstable subjects as in cases where there is no offspring or a loss of offspring. It underlines the need for the importance of understanding psychological angle in recurrent spontaneous miscarriages pertinently.[6]

REFERENCES

1. Bardos J, Hercz D, Friedenthal J, et al. A national survey on public perceptions of miscarriage. Obstet Gynecol. 2015;125(6):1313-20.
2. Zhang YX, Zhang XQ, Wang QR, et al. Psychological burden, sexual satisfaction and erectile function in men whose partners experience recurrent pregnancy loss in China: a cross-sectional study. Reprod Health. 2016;13(1):73.
3. Berle BB, Javert CT. Stress and habitual miscarriage: their relationship and the effect of therapy. Obstet Gynecol. 1954;3(3):298-306.
4. Grimm ER. Psychological investigations of habitual miscarriages. Psychom Med. 1962;24:369-78.

5. Hall RC, Beresford TP, Quinones JE. Grief following spontaneous miscarriage. Psychiatric Clin North Am. 1987;10:405-20.
6. Javert CT, Finn WF, Stander JH. Primary and secondary habitual miscarriage. Am J Obstet Gynecol. 1949;57:878-89.
7. Reinharz S. What's missing in miscarriage? J Commun Psychol. 1988;16(1):84-103.
8. Simon NM, Rothman D, Goff JT, et al. Psychological factors related to spontaneous and therapeutic abortion. Am J Obstet Gynecol. 1969;104(6):799-808.
9. Andalib A, Rezaie A, Oreizy F, et al. A study on stress, depression and NK cytotoxic potential in women with recurrent spontaneous abortion. Iran J Allergy Asthma Immunol. 2006;5(1):9-16.
10. Kolte AM, Olsen LR, Mikkelsen EM, et al. Depression and emotional stress is highly prevalent among women with recurrent pregnancy loss. Hum Reprod. 2015;30(4):777-82.
11. Hori S, Nakano Y, Furukawa TA, et al. Psychosocial factors regulating natural-killer cell activity in recurrent spontaneous abortions. Am J Reprod Immunol. 2000;44(5):299-302.
12. Sugiura-Ogasawara M, Furukawa TA, Nakano Y, et al. Depression as a potential causal factor in subsequent miscarriage in recurrent spontaneous aborters. Hum Reprod. 2002;17(10):2580-4.
13. Brost L, Kenny JW. Pregnancy after perinatal loss: parental reactions and nursing interventions. J Obstet Gynecol Neonatal Nurs. 1992;21(6):457-63.
14. Condon JT. Prevention of emotional disability following stillbirth—the role of the obstetric team. Aust N Z J Obstet Gynaecol. 1987;27(4):323-9.
15. Hall RC, Beresford TP, Quinones JE. Grief following spontaneous miscarriage. Psychiatric Clin North Am. 1987;10:405-20.
16. Stirtzinger R, Robinson GE. The psychologic effects of spontaneous abortion. CMAJ. 1989;140(7):799-801.

Chapter 10

Evidence-based Practice in Recurrent Spontaneous Miscarriages

INTRODUCTION

Any concept in clinical practice holds credibility if there is enough evidence to support the same. The term was originally used to describe an approach to teaching the practice of medicine and improving decisions by individual physicians about individual patients.[1] In fact, the entire concept of "evidence-based practice" in medical sciences is the contribution of obstetrics to the medical world. Dr Murray Enkin, Dr Iain Chalmers, and Dr Marc Kearse pioneered an effort during the 1980s and early 1990s to develop the largest database of controlled trials in medicine, as it applies to pregnancy and childbirth care. It was then used to generate some systematic reviews and recommended changes in practice standards which have changed the face of practice. These innovations led directly to the development of the Cochrane Collaboration within which this model of "evidence-based medicine" has been adopted by many other specialties.[1]

CLASSIFICATION OF EVIDENCE LEVELS

Evidence can be of wide variety and types. Evidence can be vague, can be based on randomized controlled trials (RCTs), or based on observer evidence. It is, therefore, necessary to understand what we exactly mean by a particular type of evidence. This is for reason of uniformity, scientific comparison, and drawing valid conclusions. The most commonly used evidence levels are:[2]

- *Evidence level I:* These are the best. They are further classified as:
  - Ia evidence obtained from meta-analysis of RCTs.
  - Ib evidence obtained from at least one RCT.
- *Evidence level II:*
  - IIa evidence obtained from at least one well-designed controlled study without randomization.
  - IIb evidence obtained from at least one other type of well-designed quasi-experimental study.
- *Evidence level III:*
  - III evidence obtained from well-designed nonexperimental descriptive studies, such as comparative studies, correlation studies, and case studies.
- *Evidence level IV:*
  - IV evidence obtained from expert committee reports or opinions and/or clinical experience of respected authorities.

Grades of Recommendations

On the basis of the level of evidence different scientific organizations evolve their recommendations. These recommendations are classified as "grades" of recommendations.

These are:
- *Grade of recommendation A:*
  - Requires at least one RCT as part of a body of literature of overall good quality and consistency addressing the specific recommendation (evidence levels IA, IB).
- *Grade of recommendation B:*
  - Requires the availability of well-controlled clinical studies but no RCT on the topic of recommendations (evidence levels IIA, IIB, and III).
- *Grade of recommendation C:*
  - Requires evidence obtained from expert committee reports or opinions and/or clinical experiences of respected authorities. It indicates an absence of directly applicable clinical Studies of Good Quality (Evidence Level IV).

    (Levels and grades of evidence-based on: Provan D, Stasi R, Newland AC, et al. International consensus report on the investigation and management of primary immune thrombocytopenia. Blood. 2010;115(2):168-86).[2]

Now let us examine different concepts in the clinical practice of recurrent spontaneous miscarriages in the light of these evidences.

GENETIC FACTORS

Grade of Recommendation C

- The finding of an abnormal parental karyotype should prompt referral to a clinical geneticist. The incidence of structural chromosome abnormalities, usually a balanced translocation is increased in couples with recurrent miscarriages. All the four factors, namely (1) Low maternal age at second miscarriage, (2) A history of three or more miscarriages, (3) A history of two or more miscarriages in a brother or sister, and (4) A history of two or more miscarriages in the parents of either partner increase the probability of carrier status. It is thus advised to refer for parental karyotype only when the likelihood of carrier status is 2.2% or more. All couples with a history of recurrent spontaneous miscarriages should have peripheral blood karyotyping performed.[3]
- While it is routine practice to send products of conception for histological examination, mainly to exclude a gestational trophoblastic disorder, the usefulness of histopathological investigation of placental, and fetal tissue on future pregnancy management for an individual couple remains to be determined.[3]

Evidence Level IV

Preimplantation genetic diagnosis as a treatment option for translocation carriers is a technically demanding procedure and experience is still limited. Since the technique necessitates that the couple undergoes in vitro fertilization (IVF) to produce embryos, couples with proven fertility need to be aware of the low implantation and live-birth rates per cycle following IVF. Further, they should be informed that they have a 40–50% chance of a healthy live birth in future untreated pregnancies following natural conception.[4]

Grade of Recommendation C

In all couples with a history of recurrent spontaneous miscarriages, cytogenetic analysis of the products of conception should be performed if the next pregnancy fails.[5]

Evidence Level IV

If the karyotype of the miscarried pregnancy is abnormal, there is a better prognosis in the next pregnancy. Cytogenetic testing is an expensive tool and may be reserved for patients who have undergone treatment in the index pregnancy.[6]

National Institute for Health and Care Excellence Guidelines

Parental chromosomal rearrangements: In approximately 2–5% of couples with recurrent miscarriage, one of the partners carries a balanced structural chromosomal anomaly: most commonly a balanced reciprocal or Robertsonian translocation.[4-7]

ANATOMICAL FACTORS

The routine use of hysterosalpingography as a screening test for uterine anomalies in women with recurrent spontaneous miscarriages is questionable. It is associated with patient discomfort, carries a risk of pelvic infection and radiation exposure, and is no more sensitive than the noninvasive two-dimensional pelvic ultrasound assessment of the uterine cavity. Since three-dimensional ultrasound offer both diagnosis and classification of uterine malformation, its use may obviate the need for diagnostic hysteroscopy and laparoscopy.[8]

Good Practice

All women with recurrent spontaneous miscarriages should have a pelvic ultrasound to assess uterine anatomy and morphology.[8]

CERVICAL WEAKNESS

Grade of Recommendation B

Cervical cerclage is associated with potential hazards related to the surgery and the risk of stimulating uterine contractions and hence should only be considered in women who are likely to benefit.[9]

Evidence Level IB

Cervical weakness is often overdiagnosed as a cause of midtrimester miscarriage. There is currently no satisfactory objective test that can identify women with cervical weakness in the nonpregnant state. The diagnosis is usually based on a history of late miscarriage, preceded by spontaneous rupture of membranes or painless cervical dilatation. Transvaginal ultrasound assessment of the cervix during pregnancy may be useful in predicting preterm birth in some cases of suspected cervical weakness. However, two RCTs failed to demonstrate any resulting significant improvement in perinatal survival from ultrasound indicated cervical cerclage. The Medical Research Council (MRC)/Royal College of Obstetricians and Gynecologists (RCOG) trial of elective cervical cerclage reported a small decrease in preterm birth and delivery of very low-birth weight babies,[9] but the benefit was most marked in women with three or more 2nd trimester miscarriages or preterm births. However, there was no significant improvement in perinatal survival.[9]

ENDOCRINAL FACTORS

- Other endocrine disorders, including hypersecretion of luteinizing hormone (LH), high androgen levels, hyperprolactinemia, and luteal phase defects (LPDs) have been associated with recurrent miscarriages. Current evidence suggests, however, that, as is the case for hypothyroidism, infertility is more likely a problem than pregnancy loss. Obesity is associated with a statistically significant increased risk of 1st trimester and recurrent spontaneous miscarriages. However, well-controlled diabetes mellitus is not a risk factor for recurrent miscarriage, nor is treated thyroid dysfunction.[10,11]

- *Good practice:* Routine screening for occult diabetes and thyroid disease with oral glucose tolerance and thyroid function tests in asymptomatic women presenting with recurrent spontaneous miscarriages is uninformative.[11]

PROGESTERONE SUPPLEMENTATION

A review of 14 RCTs (2,158 women) found no evidence that progestogens can prevent miscarriage. There was no difference in the incidence of adverse effects on either the mother or baby was apparent. There was evidence, however, that women who have suffered three or more miscarriages may benefit from progestogen during pregnancy. Four trials showed a decrease in miscarriage compared with placebo or no treatment in these women; however, the trials were of poorer methodological quality so these findings should be interpreted with caution. No differences were found between the route of administration of progestogen (oral, intramuscular, and vaginal) versus placebo or no treatment. More trials are needed and are underway to further clarify the effects in women with multiple prior miscarriages and to further clarify any impact on fetal anomalies.[12]

HUMAN CHORIONIC GONADOTROPIN SUPPLEMENTATION

A review included five randomized controlled studies, involving 596 women. When comparing the women who were treated with human chorionic gonadotropin (HCG) versus placebo or no treatment, there was a benefit in using HCG. However, when two of the older studies with weaker methodology were excluded, there was no longer evidence of benefit in using HCG for preventing recurrent miscarriages. As a result, firm recommendations could not be made. There were no documented adverse effects associated with using HCG. More good quality studies with larger sample sizes are needed to evaluate the use of HCG compared with other treatments and nonpharmacological strategies, such as early and accessible career contact and support.[13]

Grade of Recommendation B

- Prepregnancy suppression of high LH concentration among ovulatory women with recurrent spontaneous miscarriages and polycystic ovaries who hypersecrete LH does not improve the live-birth rate.[14]
- Polycystic ovary morphology itself does not predict an increased risk of future pregnancy loss among ovulatory women with a history of recurrent spontaneous miscarriages who conceive spontaneously.[14]
- There is insufficient evidence to assess the effect of hyperprolactinemia as a risk factor for recurrent spontaneous miscarriages. Also, there is a lack of evidence (from a single randomized trial with a small sample size, and judged to be at high risk of bias) to evaluate the effectiveness of dopamine agonists for preventing future miscarriage in women with idiopathic hyperprolactinemia and a history of recurrent miscarriage. Further high-quality research in this area is warranted.[14]

IMMUNE FACTORS

Grade of Recommendation B

Routine screening for thyroid antibodies in women with recurrent spontaneous miscarriages is not recommended.[15]

Grade of Recommendation A

- Currently, there is no reliable evidence to show that steroids improve the live-birth rate of women with recurrent spontaneous miscarriages associated with antiphospholipid (APL) when compared with other treatment modalities.[16] Their use may provoke significant maternal and fetal morbidity. The use of intravenous immunoglobulin (IVIG), antitumor necrosis factor-α (TNF-α), glucocorticoids, or cellular therapies to prevent or reduce an "excessive immune response" and abrogate maternal–

fetal incompatibility in women with recurrent miscarriages remains controversial.[16]
- Multiple courses of glucocorticoids during pregnancy are associated with serious side effects including an increased risk of preterm birth because of premature rupture of membranes and the development of preeclampsia and gestational diabetes.[17]
- In women with a history of recurrent spontaneous miscarriages and APL, the future live- birth rate is significantly improved when a combination therapy of aspirin plus heparin is prescribed.[17]

Grade of Recommendation B

Pregnancies associated with APL treated with aspirin and heparin remains at high risk of complications during all three trimesters.[18]

Grade of Recommendation A

Immunotherapy, including paternal cell immunization, third-party donor leukocytes, trophoblast membranes, and IVIG, in women with previous unexplained recurrent spontaneous miscarriages, does not improve the live-birth rate.[19]

INFECTIONS AND RECURRENT SPONTANEOUS ABORTION

Grade of Recommendation B

Toxoplasmosis, other (congenital syphilis and viruses), rubella, cytomegalovirus, and herpes simplex virus (TORCH) screening is unhelpful in the investigation of recurrent spontaneous miscarriages.[20]

Cochrane Review

Antibiotic treatment can eradicate bacterial vaginosis in pregnancy. The overall risk of PTB was not significantly reduced. This review provides little evidence that screening and treating all pregnant women with bacterial vaginosis will prevent PTB and its consequences.[21]

A summary of recommended investigative workup of a couple with recurrent spontaneous miscarriages is shown in Box 10.1.

Box 10.1: Recommendations for the testing of couple presenting with recurrent spontaneous miscarriages.

Basic investigations:
- Obstetric and family history, age, BMI, organic solvents, alcohol, mercury, lead, caffeine, hyperthermia, and smoking
- Full blood count (blood sugar level and thyroid function tests)
- Antiphospholipid antibodies (LAC and aCA)
- Parental karyotype (after two miscarriages)
- Pelvic ultrasound (SIS) and/or hysterosalpingogram and hysteroscopy and laparoscopy in case of inconclusive findings.

Research investigations within the context of a trial:
- Fetoplacental karyotypes
- Testing of uterine and/or peripheral blood NK cells
- Luteal phase endometrial biopsy
- Homocysteine/folic acid level
- Thrombophilia screening.

(aCA: anticardiolipin antibody; BMI: body mass index; LAC: lupus anticoagulant; NK: natural killer; SIS: saline infusion sonography)

OTHER TREATMENTS

- *Tender loving care:* A small number of nonrandomized studies have reported that psychological support, that is, tender loving care (TLC) in early pregnancy, decreases miscarriage rates in women with unexplained recurrent miscarriages.[22]
- *Vitamin supplements:* Taking any vitamin supplements prior to pregnancy or in early pregnancy does not prevent women experiencing miscarriage. However, evidence showed that women receiving multivitamins plus iron and folic acid had reduced risk for stillbirth. There is insufficient evidence to examine the effects of different combinations of vitamins on miscarriage and miscarriage-related outcomes.[23]
- *Chinese herbal medicine:* There was limited evidence (from nine studies with small sample sizes and unclear risk of bias) to assess the effectiveness of Chinese herbal medicines for treating unexplained recurrent miscarriage; no data were available

to assess the safety of the intervention for the mother or her baby. More high-quality studies are needed to further evaluate the effectiveness and safety of Chinese herbal medicines for unexplained recurrent miscarriage.[24]

- *Methyltetrahydrofolate versus folic acid:* There was no significant difference in abortion rate between two groups. Serum folate increased significantly in both groups over time; these changes were significantly higher in the group receiving 5-methyltetrahydrofolate (5- MTHF) than the group receiving folic acid, and the result was the same by considering the time.[25]

A summary of treatments recommended and otherwise for recurrent spontaneous miscarriages is shown in Box 10.2.

Box 10.2: Recommendations for the treatment of recurrent spontaneous miscarriages.

Established treatment:
- Tender loving care (TLC)
- Health advices (diet, coffee, smoking, and alcohol).

Treatment requiring more RCTs:
- Aspirin and/or heparin for women presenting with APLA or inherited thrombophilias
- Progesterone in women presenting with unexplained early and late recurrent miscarriages
- Folic acid in women presenting with hyperhomocysteinemia.

Treatment with no proven benefits:
- Immunization with paternal leukocytes or trophoblast membranes.

Treatment associated with more harm than good
- Daily corticosteroids during first half of pregnancy.

(APLA: antiphospholipid antibody; RCTs: randomized controlled trials)

ALLIED ASPECTS

In allied aspects, some common practices associated with miscarriages have been reviewed and conclusions are as follows:

- *Bed rest during pregnancy for preventing miscarriage:*
  - *Not enough evidence to say if bed rest helps in preventing miscarriage:* A review of two trials, involving 84 women, found that there was not sufficient evidence from high-

quality studies to be able to say whether bed rest helps to prevent miscarriage or not. Care for women at increased risk of miscarriage needs to be offered according to their individual needs.[26]

- *Comparing medical treatments for miscarriage with waiting for nature to take its course or using surgery to empty the womb:*
  - The available evidence suggests that medical treatment, with misoprostol, and expectant care are both acceptable alternatives to routine surgical evacuation given the availability of health service resources to support all three approaches. Further studies, including long-term follow-up, are needed to confirm these findings.[27]
- *Surgical removal of fibroids does not improve fertility outcomes:*
  - One review included three studies with 474 participants and aimed to answer two questions. Firstly, whether myomectomy led to an improvement in fertility, and secondly if the procedure is beneficial, what is the ideal surgical approach. Only one study was found that examined the effect of myomectomy on fertility and it found no significant benefit. However, there are some concerns regarding how the data were analyzed, and therefore, the evidence cannot be considered to be conclusive until further studies are available. Only two studies have been identified relating to the choice of the surgical approach to the myomectomy. They compared open versus laparoscopic myomectomy and found no difference in fertility outcomes. Therefore, again more studies are needed before a definite conclusion can be reached.[28]

REFERENCES

1. Evidence-Based Medicine Working Group. Evidence-based medicine. A new approach to teaching the practice of medicine. JAMA. 1992;268(17):2420-5.
2. Provan D, Stasi R, Newland AC, et al. International consensus report on the investigation and management of primary immune thrombocytopenia. Blood. 2010;115(2):168-86.
3. Desai P. Recurrent Spontaneous Miscarriages, 2nd edition. New Delhi: Jaypee Brothers Medical Publishers (P) Ltd; 2014. pp. 116-7.

4. De Braekeleer M, Dao TN. Cytogenetic studies in couples experiencing repeated pregnancy losses. Hum Reprod. 1990;5(5):519-28.
5. Clifford K, Rai R, Watson H, et al. An informative protocol for the investigation of recurrent miscarriage: preliminary experience of 500 consecutive cases. Hum Reprod. 1994;9(7):1328-32.
6. Stephenson MD, Sierra S. Reproductive outcomes in recurrent pregnancy loss associated with a parental carrier of a structural chromosome rearrangement. Hum Reprod. 2006;21(4):1076-82.
7. Franssen MT, Korevaar JC, van der Veen F, et al. Reproductive outcome after chromosome analysis in couples with two or more miscarriages: index [corrected]-control study. BMJ. 2006;332(7544):759-63.
8. Royal College of Obstetricians and Gynecologists (RCOG). (2011). The Investigation and Treatment of Couples with Recurrent First-trimester and Second-trimester Miscarriage: Green-top Guideline No. 17. [online] Available from www.rcog.org.uk/globalassets/documents/guidelines/gtg_17.pdf. [Accessed October, 2017].
9. Interim report of the Medical Research Council/Royal College of Obstetricians and Gynaecologists multicentre randomized trial of cervical cerclage. MRC/RCOG Working Party on Cervical Cerclage. Br J Obstet Gynaecol. 1988;95(5):437-45.
10. Mills JL, Simpson JL, Driscoll SG, et al. Incidence of spontaneous abortion among normal women and insulin-dependent diabetic women whose pregnancies were identified within 21 days of conception. N Engl J Med. 1988;319(25):1617-23.
11. Abalovich M, Gutierrez S, Alcaraz G, et al. Overt and subclinical hypothyroidism complicating pregnancy. Thyroid. 2002;12(1):63-8.
12. Haas DM, Ramsey PS. Progestogen for preventing miscarriage. Cochrane Database Syst Rev. 2013;(10):CD003511.
13. Morley LC, Simpson N, Tang T. Human chorionic gonadotrophin (hCG) for preventing miscarriage. Cochrane Database Syst Rev. 2013;(1):CD008611.
14. Chen H, Fu J, Huang W. Dopamine agonists for preventing future miscarriage in women with idiopathic hyperprolactinemia and recurrent miscarriage history. Cochrane Database Syst Rev. 2016;(7):CD008883.
15. Abbassi-Ghanavati M. Thyroid autoantibodies and pregnancy outcomes. Clin Obstet Gynecol. 2011;54(3):499-505.
16. Jeve YB, Davies W. Evidence-based management of recurrent miscarriages. J Hum Reprod Sci. 2014;7(3):159-69.
17. Murphy KE, Hannah ME, Willan AR, et al. Maternal side-effects after multiple courses of antenatal corticosteroids (MACS): the three-month follow-up of women in the randomized controlled trial of MACS for preterm birth study. J Obstet Gynaecol Can. 2011;33(9):909-21.

18. Simcox LE, Ormesher L, Tower C, et al. Thrombophilia and pregnancy complications. Int J Mol Sci. 2015;16(12):28418-28.
19. Pundir J, Coomaraswami A. Gynecology Evidence-based Algorithms, 1st edition. Cambridge: Cambridge University press; 2016. p. 14.
20. Regan L, Jivraj S. Infection and pregnancy loss. In: MacLean AB, Regan L, Carrington D (Eds). Infection and Pregnancy. London: RCOG Press; 2001. pp. 291-304.
21. Brocklehurst P, Gordon A, Heatley E, et al. Antibiotics for treating bacterial vaginosis in pregnancy. Cochrane Database Syst Rev. 2013;(1):CD000262.
22. Jauniaux E, Farquharson RG, Christiansen OB, et al. Evidence-based guidelines for the investigation and medical treatment of recurrent miscarriage. Hum Reprod. 2006;21(9):2216-22.
23. Balogun OO, da Silva Lopes K, Ota E, et al. Vitamin supplementation for preventing miscarriage. Cochrane Database Syst Rev. 2016;(5): CD004073.
24. Li L, Dou L, Leung PC, et al. Chinese herbal medicines for unexplained recurrent miscarriage. Cochrane Database Syst Rev. 2016;(1):CD010568.
25. Hekmatdoost A, Vahid F, Yari Z, et al. Methyltetrahydrofolate vs Folic Acid Supplementation in Idiopathic Recurrent Miscarriage with Respect to Methylenetetrahydrofolate Reductase C677T and A1298C Polymorphisms: A Randomized Controlled Trial. PLoS One. 2015;10(12):e0143569.
26. Aleman A, Althabe F, Belizán J, et al. Bed rest during pregnancy for preventing miscarriage. Cochrane Database Syst Rev. 2005;(2): CD003576.
27. Kim C, Barnard S, Neilson JP, et al. Medical treatments for incomplete miscarriage. Cochrane Database Syst Rev. 2017;(1):CD007223.
28. Metwally M, Cheong YC, Horne AW. Surgical treatment of fibroids for subfertility. Cochrane Database Syst Rev. 2012;(11):CD003857.

Chapter 11

Approach to a Subject with Recurrent Spontaneous Miscarriages

INTRODUCTION

Recurrent spontaneous miscarriage is interlinked with many other obstetric vasculopathies. As a result, when we approach a subject with this condition it will be necessary to remember that close surveillance will not end at 12–14 weeks but will continue till term. While a subject may not have a recurrent miscarriage this time but she can have preeclampsia or intrauterine growth restriction (IUGR) or a stillbirth. It is because all vasculopathies are interlinked.

There is a fragile line that segregates one cause of recurrent spontaneous miscarriage from the other. A patient interaction with the subject helps the obstetrician in separating one cause from the other. More precise the diagnoses better the results. It will also be necessary to remember that in many couples different causes operate in different pregnancies. A keen clinical sense, therefore, will be of great help in differentiating one cause from the other.

THE FIRST CONSULTATION

It is desirable to have the first consultation with the obstetrician in the interval period when the subject is not pregnant. The first step at this meeting will be to differentiate between a miscarriage and a delayed period. In many subjects delayed periods get wrongly labeled as pregnancy. On nearly all occasions these so-called pregnancies are never confirmed by a doctor. These are usually anovulatory subjects who get bunched in the group of recurrent miscarriages. Many times subjects with polycystic ovarian syndrome (PCOS) tend to have a false-positive pregnancy test. A discerning doctor can easily differentiate a false-positive test of a PCOS from a genuinely positive test. The problem arises when the subject performs a home pregnancy test and interprets it as a positive test which in reality could be a false-positive test. This false-positive pregnancy test is due to the cross-reactivity of luteinizing hormone (LH) with human chorionic gonadotropin (HCG). Some newer urinary pregnancy tests have apparently tackled this problem to a great extent.

Once the obstetrician has confirmed that these were recurrent miscarriages he should approach the subject very systematically. It is important to study from her records as at what weeks of gestation did these miscarriages occur?

Miscarriages: At what weeks?

This clinical investigation will significantly help the obstetrician to differentiate some causes from one another. Miscarriages in early weeks (up to 8 weeks) are usually of genetic cause. Also, in subjects with other features of PCOS these early miscarriages could be due to this endocrinal cause. Late miscarriages—meaning miscarriages occurring in late 1st trimester or early 2nd trimester are usually immunological and due to rare causes like hyperhomocysteinemia.

Conceptus Alive or Fetal Demise at Miscarriage

A critical lead question as to whether these were live miscarriages or fetal demises (missed abortions as was known in the past) is necessary. A live conceptus getting miscarried suggests an anatomical cause. Usually, these are during later weeks of pregnancy in 2nd trimester. If there was a fetal or embryonic demise, then the weeks at which it occurred become important. Embryonic demise at early weeks of pregnancy (less than 8 weeks) suggests a germ-cell defect or an endocrinal cause. Fetal demise in late 1st trimester or early 2nd trimester suggests an immunological cause. There can be some overlap in the periods of miscarriages. Nevertheless, a broad picture can be conceptualized in the mind of the clinician by getting this vital information.

With the earlier information, any good clinician can get a reasonable idea of the etiology. The question now arises is: what are the laboratory investigations which need to be carried out? It needs to be stressed that laboratory studies may or may not be very helpful in subjects with recurrent miscarriages. Therefore, a solid clinical acumen to diagnose the cause of miscarriage is vital. Also, there are some causes where laboratory investigations may not be available as yet. The classic example of this is miscarriages due to an alloimmune cause. There are investigations like antiphospholipid antibodies (APLAs) for autoimmune causes of recurrent miscarriages, but there are no investigations for alloimmune causes. Also among autoimmune causes, there are many antibodies which are known to science but are still not viable for the laboratories to test. Thus, they are known to exist but may not be picked up on laboratory investigations. For autoimmune causes of recurrent miscarriages, therefore, APLA testing suffices. There is no need to test for antinuclear (ANA) antibodies. For endocrinal causes relevant investigations for PCOS including those for insulin resistance and follicle-stimulating hormone (FSH):LH ratio will be of help. Karyotyping of the parents or chromosomal study of the products of conception miscarried have their limitations which are discussed in the chapter on Genetics of Recurrent Miscarriages and Other Pregnancy Losses of this book. Thus, relevant laboratory investigations can be tailored to the need.

As it has been made amply clear in this book, in the chapter Infections and Recurrent Spontaneous Miscarriages, testing for toxoplasmosis, other (congenital syphilis and viruses), rubella, cytomegalovirus, and herpes simplex virus (TORCH) infections is not necessary and should be discontinued forthwith. Thankfully since the publishing of the previous edition of this book TORCH testing has reduced in subjects with recurrent spontaneous miscarriages, however, many clinicians are still requesting this investigation. This practice should be immediately discontinued.

Associated Features

A sharp clinical observation skill also helps the obstetrician to approach a subject with recurrent miscarriages productively. Features of insulin resistance like central obesity or a faint line of hirsutism on the upper lip can give a clue to the endocrinal cause in this subject. A history of seemingly diverse conditions like stillbirth or accidental hemorrhage should give away the immunological causes causing losses in these subjects. It can avoid unnecessary investigations and also make the management of the couple more professional.

It is not uncommon to see a chromosomal evaluation of couples with recurrent miscarriages. It is an entirely rational practice, but an average obstetrician finds it difficult to handle the reports. A presence of 5% cells that exhibit some form of mosaicism in the mother may not have any significance if there are no associated features that have manifested. It is, therefore, mandatory for the obstetrician to request this investigation only after a sound interpretation has been learned or the interpretation should be left to the geneticist. It should be acknowledged that the genetic laboratories usually give a detailed report and even the limitations as well as the possible interpretations. However, in clinical practice, it is often found that even a small abnormality may be latched onto by the obstetrician. The couple is then made to believe that it is "genetically" wrong and so is losing babies repeatedly.

Reassurance is Critical

Reassurance is the first step to tender loving care in subjects with recurrent spontaneous miscarriages. Many times we encounter couples who tell that the treating doctor did not listen to them properly and was in a great hurry to prescribe. It is imperative for an obstetrician to be prepared to invest in his patients in the form of time. If an obstetrician does not have enough time for his subjects with recurrent spontaneous miscarriages, his results will be suboptimal. A proper explanation is the key. It will be wrong to say to a subject who is expressing her grief that we understand what she is undergoing. No one understands what she endures except herself. At the most, the obstetrician can have empathy for her. It is also necessary for the obstetrician to allow her to grieve. These subjects weep and express great exasperation when they come for consultation. It is necessary for us to allow her to grieve. Many times obstetricians stop them from crying or cut short her expression of exasperation. It should not be done.

It is also necessary for the obstetrician to tell her clear chances of spontaneous resolution. At any given instance of time after recurrent miscarriages, there is a 70% chance of spontaneous resolution. The couple gets great morale boost when this scientific information is shared with them. They see a hope and instantly collect themselves to brace up for the next pregnancy.

The natural question that follows is how long they should wait for the next conception? The answer in most situations should be there is no need to wait once she is medically fit. It means her hemoglobin status should be corrected if there is anemia. If there is an endocrinal cause that needs to be treated. Her emotional stability should be restored. Once the cause and the effects of previously failed pregnancy are taken care of, she can plan a pregnancy. Needless to add, as soon as she plans a pregnancy she should start folic acid 5 mg per day preconception. If there is an immunological cause, she has to start aspirin as described in the chapter on Immunological Causes of Recurrent Miscarriages.

ON CONCEPTION

First visit postconception should be as early as possible. Once the patient misses her period, she will visit the obstetrician. At this time all her reports must be reviewed once again. Clinical symptoms and signs of pregnancy will be very useful to infer if the conceptus is alive. It is a good friend of the obstetrician as it is reassuring even without a sonography. The patient must also be informed that these are good signs and her conceptus is alive.

Ultrasonography on the first visit is very important. Besides other vital leads, it confirms the pregnancy, estimates the period of gestation, and registers cardiac activity if seen. Features like chorionic density, its uniformity, and presence or absence of subchorionic hemorrhage also need to be noted. Yolk sac in the gestational sac within the uterus does not give any great information except for the fact that it confirms an intrauterine pregnancy. If large yolk sac is seen, the prognosis is not very good. Also, unusual features in the yolk sac like double yolk sac may vaguely hint at a malformed fetus. All these features are of secondary help in the subject with recurrent spontaneous miscarriages.

The approach to be followed after that is as per the cause identified and has been detailed in each chapter in much greater depth.

Index

Page numbers followed by *b* refer to box, *f* refer to figure, and *t* refer to table.

A

Aborters
  primary 55
  secondary 55
Abortion, threatened 54
Acquired uterine anomalies 28
Activated partial thromboplastin
    time 70
Adverse pregnancy outcomes 116
AES *See* Androgen excess society
AFI *See* Amniotic fluid index
Allograft inflammatory factor-1 46
American Fertility Society 21, 23*b*
Amniotic fluid index 8*f*
Androgen Excess Society 107
Anembryonic pregnancy 16
Anemia 152
Antibiotic treatment 142
Anticardiolipin 57
  antibody 68, 143
Antinuclear antibodies, test for 150
Antiphospholipid antibody 56, 61,
    126, 144, 150
  originating in infections 126
Antiphospholipid
  prevalence of 58
  syndrome 56, 86
APA syndrome, treatment of 69
APL syndrome *See* Antiphospholipid
    syndrome
APLA *See* Antiphospholipid
    antibody
APTT *See* Activated partial
    thromboplastin time
Arcuate uterus 27
Asherman's syndrome 31
Aspirin plus heparin therapy 72
Aspirin/heparin 71
Assisted reproductive technology 31
  program 81
Autopsy 87
  virtual 87

B

Bacterial vaginosis 122, 124
Beta human chorionic gonadotropin
    10
Bicornuate uterus 25
  complete 26
  pregnancy in 38*f*
  USG of 26*f*
Blighted ovum 81
BMI *See* Body mass index
Body mass index 143
Body's immune response 117

C

Cadherins 62
Calcium-dependent adhesion 62
Cardiac activity 12*f*
  absent 13*f*
  positive 6
Cardiac motion, detecting 9
Cardiotocography 7, 9*f*
Central nervous system 83
Cerebral artery, middle 7, 8*f*
Cervical
  cerclage 34, 102
  incompetence 31
    diagnosis of 32
  weakness 139
Cesarean section, lower segment 36,
    37*f*, 38*f*

Chimerism 80
Chinese herbal medicine 143
Chlamydia trachomatis 122, 124
Chromosomal abnormalities 84
   high risk for 85
   in abortuses 82t
Chromosomal anomalies 84
   in abortuses 82t
   in parents 78
   in perinatal deaths, frequency of 83t
Chromosomal rearrangements, types of 83t
CNS *See* Central nervous system
Collin's knife 24
Conceptus alive 149
Congenital abnormalities 102
Congenital syphilis 142, 150
Congenital uterine anomalies 17, 22
   diagnosis of 21
Corpus luteum flow 16
Coxiella burnetii 125
Cushing's syndrome 107
Cystathionine beta-synthase 43
Cystic fibrosis transmembrane conductance regulator 78
Cytochrome 105
Cytokines 116
   protective 6
   types of 6
Cytomegalovirus 121, 122, 150

D

DES *See* Diethylstilbestrol
Destructive cytokines 6
Diabetes 95
Didelphys 23
Diethylstilbestrol 18t
   exposure-related anomalies 28
Doppler findings 16
Doppler in early pregnancy loss, qualitative observations on 16t
Dydrogesterone 102
Dysmenorrhea 17

E

Early fetal loss and malformation 86b
Early pregnancy failure, diagnosing 4
Ectopic pregnancy 26
Efficient syncytiotrophoblasts system 66
Embryo 45
Embryonic demise 16
   radiographic assessment of 10b
Embryonic heart rate 10
Embryonic tissues 80
Endocrinal factors 139
Endometrial cavities, separate 24f
Endometriosis 115
   causes of 117
Endometrium, benign growths from 28
Endoscopy 20
European Society for Gynecological Endoscopy Consensus on Diagnosis 18
European Society of Human Reproduction and Embryology 18

F

Female genital anomalies 18
Fetal
   autopsy 87
   cardiac activity 9
   demise
      at miscarriage 149
      ultrasonographic features of 4
   growth restriction 26
   heart rate 11t
   loss, etiological causes of 88
   malformations 84
   medicine expert 90
   microchimerism, phenomenon of 48
   pathology workups 87

Index

pole, absent 109f
tissue 88
  sampling for genetic evaluation 88
  sampling techniques 89b
  trophoblasts 49
Fetus
  as allograft 44
  as unique allograft 47
Fluorescent polymerase chain reaction, quantitative 89
Folic acid 43, 144
Follicle-stimulating hormone 103, 150

G

G protein-coupled estrogen receptor 117f
Genetic causes, investigative workup for 85
Genetic counseling 90
Genetic factors 137
  in pregnancy loss, etiologies of 78b
Genital mycoplasma 125
Gestational age 11t, 13f, 14f
Gestational sac 4
  irregular 14f
Glucocorticoids 141
GnRH See Gonadotropin-releasing hormone
Gonadotropin-releasing hormone 63
GPER See G protein-coupled estrogen receptor
Graft-versus-host diseases 48
Granulocyte-macrophage colony-stimulating factor 46

H

hCG See Human chorionic gonadotropin
Heart
  activity, absent 111f
  rate, slow 110f

Hematoxylin 87
Hemochorial pregnancy 45
Heparin 70
  earlier, discontinue 71
  side effect of 71
HER See Embryonic heart rate
Herpes simplex 122
  virus 121
  infections 150
Histocompatibility complex 45
HIV See Human immunodeficiency virus
Homocysteine 43
Human chorionic gonadotropin 15, 81, 98, 140, 149
  immunological basis of 99
  supplementation 140
Human immunodeficiency virus 121, 122
Human leukocyte antigen 47
Human menopausal gonadotropin 104
Human T-lymphotropic virus 121
Hydatidiform mole, partial 79
Hyperhomocysteinemia 43
Hyperprolactinemia 94
Hypersensitivity cells, delayed-type 55
Hypertension, chronic 66
Hypoimmunogenic embryo 47
Hysterosalpingo-contrast sonography 19
Hysterosalpingography 18
Hysteroscopy 20

I

Immune factors 141
Immunology 130
Immunomodulatory effects 73
Implantation failure 81
In vitro fertilization 69, 104, 137
  embryo transfer 92
  failures 78

Incompetent gonadotropin-releasing hormone activity 63
Infection 121, 142
   specific 124
Infertility 3
Insulin resistance 106
   severe 107
Interleukin 46
Intrauterine
   adhesions 31
   growth restriction 12, 42, 148
   synechia 31
Intravenous immunoglobulin 72, 141
IUGRs *See* Intrauterine growth retardations
IVF *See* In vitro fertilization

L

LAC *See* Lupus anticoagulant
Laparoscopic encerclage 35
Leukocyte transfusions 72
LH-releasing hormone 105
Listeria monocytogenes 122
Living organism 1
Lupus anticoagulant 143
Luteal phase defect 97, 139
   and recurrent miscarriages 97
Luteinizing hormone 2, 139
   endocrinopathy 103
   hypersecretion of 94
   suppression of 105

M

Male hormones 103
Maternal lymphatic systems 45
Maternal lymphomyeloid cells 47
Maternal protector systems and pregnancy, paralysis of 46
MCA *See* Middle cerebral artery
Medicine, evidence-based 135
Messenger ribonucleic acid 46
Methionine synthase 43
Methylenetetrahydrofolate 43
Methyltetrahydrofolate 144
Micro ribonucleic acid 117
Miracle of paradox 67
Miscarriage 3, 26, 77, 102
   early 81
   increased risk of 27
   medical treatments for 145
   partner specificity in 54
   post-treatment 25
Missed abortion 1, 81, 149
Müllerian abnormalities 17
Müllerian anomalies 23
Müllerian duct 23, 27
   anomalies 25
   malformations 22
Müllerian fusion 25
Mycoplasma hominis 122, 125
Myometrium, benign growths from 28

N

National Institute for Health and Care Excellence Guidelines 138
Natural killer cell 53, 118, 130, 143
Neodymium-doped yttrium aluminum garnet 24
Neonatal intensive care unit 37
Neural tube defect 79
NICU *See* Neonatal intensive care unit
Nitric oxide synthase 2 46
NK cell *See* Natural killer cell
Nonfertile menstrual cycle 97
Nonimmunological basis 55

O

Obstetric vasculopathy 2, 42, 44
   manifestation of 42
Oocytes, abnormalities in 78
Oogenesis, abnormal 78
Organisms associated with spontaneous miscarriages 122*t*

Index

Ovarian hyperstimulation syndrome 99
Oxygen species, reactive 80

P

Parental chromosomal rearrangements 138
Parental karyotyping 90
PCOS *See* Polycystic ovarian syndrome
PIH *See* Pregnancy-induced hypertension
Placenta 53, 80
   and cord, normal 12*f*
   protective mechanisms in 53
Placental abruption 43
Platelets 59
Polycystic ovary 111*f*
   syndrome 94, 106, 107, 107*t*, 149
Polymerase chain reaction 124
Poor prognostic indicators 10
Postzygotic
   abnormalities 79
   mitotic divisions 79
Preeclampsia 42
Pregnancy
   abnormal 16
   eight weeks 110*f*
   loss 17, 77, 115
      causes of 117
   nine weeks 111*f*
   seven weeks of 7*f*
   six weeks 109*f*
   test, false-positive 149
   with gestational sac, abnormal 4
Pregnancy-induced hypertension 12, 50
Preimplantation genetic diagnosis 89, 92
Premature rupture of membranes 122
Preterm births, prevent 102
Preterm delivery 17

Preterm labor 17, 26
   symptoms of 33
Progesterone 72, 101
   and human chorionic gonadotropins supplementation 98
   and recurrent spontaneous miscarriages 96
   levels, low 96
   receptor modulator 30
   supplementation 140
Protects fetus 45
Protein 116
   C activation 60
Proximal cervix, funneling of 33f
Psychology 130
Psychotherapist 133
Pyridoxine 43

R

Randomized controlled trials 135, 144
RCTs *See* Randomized controlled trials
Recurrent early pregnancy loss 96
Recurrent miscarriage 43, 96
   corticosteroids in 69
   genetic of 77
   psychological bearings of 129
Recurrent pregnancy loss 81, 85, 106, 121, 122, 124, 130, 131
   autoimmunity in 56
   specific organism and 123
   women with 22
Recurrent pregnancy miscarriage, immunology of 42
Recurrent spontaneous abortion 44, 104, 142
   causes of 44
Recurrent spontaneous miscarriage 1, 2, 65, 95, 103, 115, 121, 143*b*, 148
   anatomical causes of 17

endocrinal causes of 94
evidence-based practice in 135
management of 132
treatment of 98, 144*b*
Robotic encerclage 35
RPL *See* Recurrent pregnancy loss
Rubella 121, 122

S

Saline infusion sonography 143
Segmental müllerian agenesis-hypoplasia 23
Septate uterus 23
Sildenafil 73
Singleton versus twins 33
SIS *See* Saline infusion sonography
SLE *See* Systemic lupus erythematosus
Spermatogenesis, abnormal 79
Spontaneous resolution 65
Stillbirth 83
   and neonatal deaths 81
Strassman metroplasty 26
Subchorionic hemorrhage 6, 109
   absence of 153
   diffuse areas of 14*f*, 109*f*
   presence of 153
Subclinical hyperthyroidism 96
Submucous fibroids 29*f*
Superoxide anion radical 80
Syncytiotrophoblasts
   defective generation of 62
   privileged status of 63
Syndromes 84
Systemic lupus erythematosus 44

T

TAS *See* Transabdominal sonography
Tender loving care 131, 143
Teratogens and environmental factors 80
Testosterone 103

Three-dimensional ultrasonography 19
Thrombomodulin 60
Thromboxane prostacyclin
   mechanism, disruption of 60
Thyroid
   abnormalities 95
   function 95
TORCH 121, 142
Toxoplasmosis 121
Transabdominal sonography 5
Transforming growth factor-beta 52
Transvaginal sonography 5
Trophoblastic flow 16
Tumor necrosis factor-alpha 46
Two well-formed cervices 36*f*
Two-dimensional ultrasonography 19

U

Unicornuate 23
   uterus 26
Ureaplasma
   infection 125
   urealyticum 122, 125
Uterine
   anomalies
      classification of 18*f*
      screening test for 138
   artery
      embolization 30
      pulsatility index 61
   corpus 27
   fibroids 28
   malformation, classification of 138
   septa 23
   wall thickness 21
Uterus 53
   anatomical defects in 3
   coronal section of 24*f*
   didelphys 27
      ultrasonography of 36*f*
      intraoperative appearance of 38*f*

left 36*f*
right 36*f*

Vaginal progesterone 102
Viruses 142, 150
Vitamin 43
   B6 43
   supplements 143

Waddlia chondrophila 126
White blood cell 122, 130

Yolk sac 14
   double 15*f*

Zona pellucida 46